Register Now f[...]
to You[...]

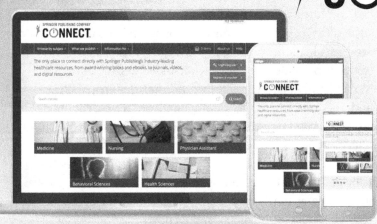

Your print purchase of *Health Services Research and Analytics Using Excel®*
includes online access to the contents of your book—increasing accessibility,
portability, and searchability!

Access today at:

**http://connect.springerpub.com/content/book/978-0-8261-5028-8
or scan the QR code at the right with your smartphone
and enter the access code below.**

25T3D0H3

*Scan here for
quick access.*

SPRINGER PUBLISHING COMPANY
View all our products at springerpub.com

Nalin Johri, PhD, MPH, MA (Social Work) is an assistant professor and assessment coordinator in the Masters in Healthcare Administration (MHA) program/Department of Interprofessional Health Sciences and Healthcare Administration/School of Health and Medical Sciences at Seton Hall University and teaches several courses, including research methods, healthcare data analytics, 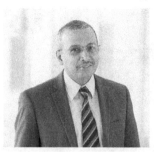 healthcare economics, healthcare policy, and financial management. His areas of interest include program evaluation, competency-based assessment, and training. Dr. Johri is a frequent presenter on competency-based assessment at the Association of University Programs in Healthcare Administration (AUPHA) Annual Meetings and was invited by the Commission on Accreditation of Healthcare Management Education (CAHME) for a national webinar. Dr. Johri's work experience includes program development, monitoring, and evaluation experience on maternal and child health and nutrition and prevention of mother-to-child transmission of HIV. His experience spans over 10 years with nongovernmental organizations such as CARE and EngenderHealth, Francois-Xavier Bagnoud Center at the University of Medicine and Dentistry of New Jersey as well as consulting with UNICEF. Until April 2013 he was the Impact Evaluation Advisor for USAID's Palestinian Health Sector Reform Project. He holds a master's degree in social work from the Tata Institute of Social Sciences, Mumbai, India, a master's degree in public health (MPH) from Emory University, and a PhD in health policy and administration from the University of North Carolina at Chapel Hill.

HEALTH SERVICES RESEARCH AND ANALYTICS USING EXCEL®

Nalin Johri, PhD, MPH, MA (Social Work)

Assistant Professor
School of Health and Medical Sciences
Seton Hall University
Nutley, New Jersey

SPRINGER PUBLISHING COMPANY

Health Services Research and Analytics Using Excel® is an independent publication and is neither affiliated with, nor authorized, sponsored, or approved by, Microsoft Corporation. Excel® is a registered trademark of the Microsoft Corporation.

Springer Publishing Company, LLC
11 West 42nd Street
New York, NY 10036
www.springerpub.com
http://connect.springerpub.com/home

Acquisitions Editor: David D'Addona
Compositor: diacriTech

ISBN: 978-0-8261-5027-1
ebook ISBN: 978-0-8261-5028-8
DOI: 10.1891/9780826150288

Qualified instructors may request supplements by emailing textbook@springerpub.com
Instructor's Manual: 978-0-8261-5036-3
Instructor's Test Bank: 978-0-8261-5037-0
Instructor's PowerPoints: 978-0-8261-5038-7

20 21 22 23 / 5 4 3 2 1

The author and the publisher of this Work have made every effort to use sources believed to be reliable to provide information that is accurate and compatible with the standards generally accepted at the time of publication. The author and publisher shall not be liable for any special, consequential, or exemplary damages resulting, in whole or in part, from the readers' use of, or reliance on, the information contained in this book. The publisher has no responsibility for the persistence or accuracy of URLs for external or third-party Internet websites referred to in this publication and does not guarantee that any content on such websites is, or will remain, accurate or appropriate.

Library of Congress Cataloging-in-Publication Data
LCCN: 2019919433

Contact us to receive discount rates on bulk purchases. We can also customize our books to meet your needs.
For more information please contact: sales@springerpub.com

Nalin Johri: https://orcid.org/0000-0002-2615-8856

Publisher's Note: **New and used products purchased from third-party sellers are not guaranteed for quality, authenticity, or access to any included digital components.**

Printed in the United States of America.

To the many teachers who have taught me to give; my students and colleagues at Seton Hall University who have made me a better teacher.

To Anandhi, my wife and best friend;

To Arundhati, my daughter;

To Kamala and P. S. Ranganathan, my in-laws; and

To Shakun and Satish Johri, my parents. Thank you!

CONTENTS

PREFACE

Health Services Research and Analytics Using Excel® grew out of my years of teaching the intricacies of Healthcare Research Methods and Statistical Analysis to graduate students in healthcare administration. The goal of this course and now this book is to develop competencies in the use of quantitative and qualitative analysis as well as 3D Maps—all within Excel! This book works through real-world examples based on healthcare datasets. If you are a petrified professional, a stymied student, or an interested instructor—this book is for you.

Early in my teaching career, I supplemented my course with existing books based on teaching statistics through Excel. This was a good start, but my students found these books either too dense or too light. To bridge this gap, I developed some of my own content in Excel as well as heard from students what their needs were—use of pivot tables as well as videos explaining the analysis using Excel. Initially, I found this ironic as there are so many videos on use of Excel. However, the catch was that these available videos did not go over examples from healthcare to which the students could relate. In this period of experimentation with Excel and my course, I discovered Add-ins related to 3D Maps as well as qualitative analysis using MeaningCloud. This was my "aha moment"! Finally, I could bundle quantitative and qualitative analysis as well as 3D Maps all within Excel. No more learning (and forgetting) proprietary stand-alone software that have these individual features— nor all of them together as it is now possible in Excel.

Quantitative/Qualitative Analysis and 3D Maps

Developed from the standpoint of active learning and engagement in the real world, this textbook includes supplementary health datasets, such as Hospital Compare Assessment of Healthcare Providers and Systems (HCAHPS); historical and current National Health Expenditure; and Community Health Rankings (used with permission from University of Wisconsin Population Health Institute; County Health Rankings & Roadmaps, 2019. www.county healthrankings.org). These supplementary datasets are available for download at https://connect.springerpub.com/content/book/978-0-8261-5028-8.

In addition, the text also includes a select list of categorized sources of healthcare data in Chapter 12, List of Select Sources of Healthcare Data. This categorized list was developed as part of a Digital Humanities Seed Grant through the Center for Faculty Development at Seton Hall University. Considerations in importing and managing these data within Excel provide familiarity with the Excel environment and the data. This crucial preparatory phase leads to exploring the data and the fields and determining innovative ways to both summarize the distributions through pivot tables as well as depict this information on charts. Next, the setup, running, and interpretation correlation and regression as well as tests of hypotheses in a variety of scenarios are detailed through available health datasets. Since tests of hypotheses are based on sample data, a brief overview of sampling and research design is included.

In a first of its kind, this text provides a hands-on approach to analyzing hypothetical qualitative hospital review comments through the MeaningCloud Add-in. This qualitative analysis includes text categorization, sentiment analysis, and topic extraction. Finally, by using location fields in HCAHPS data, the ability of the 3D Maps, another Excel Add-in, to provide visualization and package the analysis through video tours is covered.

Approach to Content

This textbook uses a competency-based, application-oriented approach through a conversational style to hold the reader's hand as we walk together through the various topics. Each chapter is brief and starts with a short vignette to motivate the content and uses screen captures together with step-by-step commentary to explain the procedures undertaken in Excel. There is minimal use of statistical formulae and jargon and *no appendices* in this text—since the focus is on application and interpretation. To make the most of this textbook, the reader should make sure to use the supplementary datasets to work along the examples in the text and complete the practice problems at the end of specific chapters.

Instructor's Resources

Detailed videos of all procedures in Excel and solved practice problems together with datasets for the examples are available via separate urls provided within each respective chapter. Chapter 11, Video Tutorials and Answers to Practice Problems Using Healthcare Datasets in Excel®, includes an overview and access to all of the video content in one location. **In addition, qualified instructors may obtain access to supplementary material (Instructor's Manual, PowerPoints, and Test Bank) by emailing textbook@springerpub. com.** This supplementary material includes additional practice problems and solutions.

Who Is This Book For?

This textbook is positioned as an essential part of graduate and advanced undergraduate studies in Healthcare Research Methods and Statistical Analysis or related courses in Healthcare Administration, Public Health, and Allied Health schools and departments. To make the most of this textbook, students or healthcare professionals do not require any prerequisite skills or mastery in statistics or Excel.

Nalin Johri

ACKNOWLEDGMENTS

The idea for *Health Services Research and Analytics Using Excel®* came about in a chance meeting with David D'Addona of Springer Publishing. This was at a time when I was thinking of pulling together content for my Healthcare Research Methods and Statistical Analysis class and bemoaning the need for a comprehensive—qualitative and quantitative—application focused text on the backbone of Excel. I received steady encouragement and support for this from Annie Hewitt, my program director at Seton Hall University, who convinced me that this is doable.

It truly takes a village to pull together a book. My village is very ably supported and cherished by Anandhi, my wife, and her superhuman abilities in her professional and personal lives to make space and support me to keep plugging away at this book. I thank my daughter Arundhati who kept plying me with tea and desserts to sweeten the journey, and my in-laws Kamala and P. S. Ranganathan who kept up a constant supply of inspirational conversations and company. In all this, I also remember my parents Shakun and Satish Johri who have made me who I am today. Incidentally, my dad happened to be in the first few batches of a graduate program in statistics in the 1960s at Agra University in India. The program was so new that he was also recruited to teach in it. With this historical connection, I feel honored to be able to write this book.

Jaclyn Shultz, my assistant editor at Springer Publishing, has always been available and very understanding. I thank her for her patience. It has been a pleasure to work with her. Last, but not least: To Joseph Stubenrauch, Ragavender Mohan, and your entire team. A big thank you for sprinkling your magic in bringing this textbook alive.

Nalin Johri

INTRODUCTION TO HEALTHCARE DATA AND THE ROLE OF EXCEL®

LEARNING OBJECTIVES

- Appreciate the sources of data in healthcare
- Describe the need to use healthcare data for decision-making
- Identify elements of a comprehensive approach to data and analysis
- Understand the role of Excel® in handling data and analysis
- Discuss competency domains for research methods and analytics
- Provide an overview of content covered in this text

In this chapter, we begin with a brief understanding of the context for data in healthcare as a backdrop to the need for developing competencies in research methods and analytics encompassing a comprehensive—quantitative, qualitative, and spatial—as well as a nimble approach to capturing, working with, analyzing, and presenting data for decision-making. After providing an overview of the content of this text, this content is mapped to competency domains.

1.1 Context

Healthcare services and delivery are currently undergoing a rapid transformation and it is deluged by data (see Box 1.1). In this state of flux and the inroads from evidence-based approaches, there is a growing need for

---

Throughout the chapter supplemental content is available for the datasets and tutorial videos. Video availability is denoted with an icon. To gain access to these items, please visit the following urls:

Datasets: https://connect.springerpub.com/content/book/978-0-8261-5028-8

⊙ Tutorial Videos: https://connect.springerpub.com/content/book/978-0-8261-5028-8/chapter/ch11

BOX 1.1 NAVIGATING THE FLOOD OF DATA

Picture this. You work for a medium-sized hospital. This hospital has access to data from a variety of sources. For starters, this hospital has invested in Health Systems Informatics and has a robust electronic health record (EHR) system. Thus, it not only has digitized patient medical records but also includes "documentation of the clinical workflow and provides alerts, reminders, therapy plans, and medication orders" (Brown, Patrick, & Pasupathy, 2012, p. 15). Next, due to foresight at the planning stage of the EHR system, this hospital also has integrated its billing system with the EHR system such that the processing of bills and claims is seamless with the medical side of its business. Also, in order to be responsive to population health, this hospital keeps track of social determinants of health in the communities from which it draws its patients. Finally, as part of its commitment to patient experience, it constantly monitors Hospital Consumer Assessment of Healthcare Providers and Systems (HCAHPS) surveys (www.hcahpsonline.org). Hospitals of various sizes, at a minimum would have access to these four sources of data—EHR, billing, social determinants of health, and HCAHPS. The data points contained in these four sources are a veritable flood of data that the hospital needs to be prepared to manage and take advantage of for decision-making and quality improvement efforts.

Being cognizant of this flood of data and the need to better manage the resource-intensive environment within healthcare, in 2008, the pioneering efforts of Don Berwick, John Whittington, and Tom Nolan culminated in the Triple Aim. The Triple Aim provides a comprehensive framework for improving population health, improving the patient experience of care and reducing per capita cost (Institute for Healthcare Improvement, 2012) of care and provides healthcare managers with measures to keep track of this Triple Aim.

The Triple Aim itself grew out of an extension of the milestone report from the Institute of Medicine—*Crossing the Quality Chasm* (Institute of Medicine, 2001). In this report, the Institute of Medicine put forth the notion that rapid advances in medicine and healthcare delivery are far outpacing currently available standards, therapies, and procedures and likened the gap between what is available and what is possible as more than a gap and closer to a chasm—hence, the title of the report. In order to bridge this chasm, the expert report outlines six areas for better health of patients (one of the Triple Aims):

- Safe—reducing errors and mistakes in care
- Effective—evidence-based care

(continued)

> ### BOX 1.1 (*continued*)
>
> - Patient-centered—patient's values and needs are respected
> - Timely—minimizing delays in providing care
> - Efficient—care is not wasteful of resources
> - Equitable—care that does not vary based on patient, sociodemographic, or regional variables
>
> In response to the flood of data and frameworks such as the Triple Aim, the bounds of data that need to be measured, monitored, and acted upon have been growing rapidly. Times such as these require a "data-driven, more scientific approach to management" (Bell & Zaric, 2013, p. 1).

analyzing overwhelming amounts of data and making sense of what they imply and using this to inform decisions. Given this whirlwind, smart approaches to both capturing, working with, analyzing, and presenting data for decision-making are imperative.

The need of the hour is to have comprehensive and nimble approaches to accomplish this task. A comprehensive approach allows for addressing a variety of data (quantitative as well as qualitative), a variety of analyses (statistical, spatial, patterns, and meaning), and using a variety of approaches to present the results. Within this framework, nimbleness allows for its ready use in a variety of scenarios and settings.

1.2 Approach Advocated

This book advocates just such an approach on the backbone of Excel. First introduced in 1985, the number of users of MS Excel worldwide has grown to hundreds of millions (Iosebashvili, 2018). By bringing to the forefront the "hidden" capabilities in Excel (see Figure 1.1) using Add-ins, it is possible to undertake both a comprehensive and a nimble approach to analysis and use of data. The referenced Add-ins are free and exponentially expand the ability to work with a variety of data sources. Three add-ins are used in this book as part of a comprehensive approach—Analysis ToolPak, 3D Maps, and MeaningCloud. Details on installing these add-ins are provided in Chapter 2, Working in Excel® and Importing Healthcare Data. As the names of these add-ins suggest, Analysis ToolPak opens capabilities for undertaking a variety of statistical analyses, 3D maps provide options for spatial and geographical analysis, while MeaningCloud facilitates textual analysis. Thus, the use of these add-ins provides a seamless approach to traditional quantitative and qualitative analysis all within Excel while also opening avenues for spatial analysis.

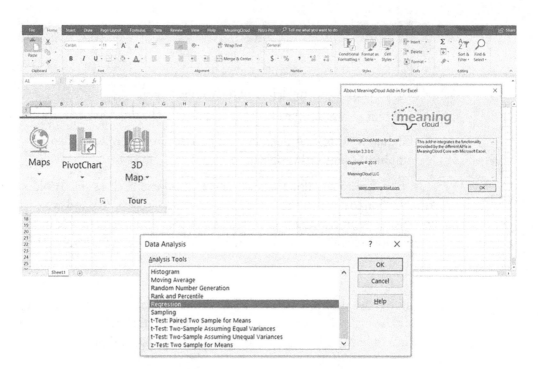

FIGURE 1.1 Data analysis, 3D maps, and MeaningCloud in Excel.

1.2.1 Available Options

There is a veritable alphabet soup of several software capable of analyzing data. In no particular order, these include SPSS, SAS, Stata, R, Python, Tableau, Epi Info™, and Excel, to name just a few. The analytical capabilities of these software are ever increasing and go together with the burgeoning need for analysts in health services. Through a comparison of the analytical capabilities of these common analytical software (Table 1.1), it is apparent that all listed software are robust in quantitative analysis capabilities, while only three (Tableau, Excel with Add-ins, and Epi Info™) include maps. However, other than Excel with the MeaningCloud Add-in, no software has available qualitative analysis capabilities. Since Excel with Add-ins provides a comprehensive approach to quantitative and qualitative analysis together with in-built maps, there is ready availability of a packaged software solution that transcends these analytical needs.

SOFTWARE	QUANTITATIVE ANALYSIS	QUALITATIVE ANALYSIS	MAPS
TABLE 1.1 Comparison of Common Software With Analytic Capabilities			
SPSS	√		
SAS	√		
Stata	√		
R	√		
Python	√		
Tableau	√		√
Epi Info™	√		√
Excel (with Add-ins)	√	√	√

1.2.2 Meeting Professional Needs

"Health services" is a professional field that is constantly evolving to address needs in a rapidly changing healthcare environment. Based on the needs in the field, accreditation requirements and the objective of professional organizations such as Commission on Accreditation of Healthcare Management Education (CAHME) and American Public Health Association (APHA) are increasingly focused on competency development, that is, not just having the knowledge but also the skills to apply this knowledge. As part of its accreditation requirements, CAHME has specific criteria (II.A, III.A, III.C, and III.D) that emphasize the need to have a competency-based model as the basis of its "curriculum, course content, learning objectives, and teaching and assessment methods" (CAHME, 2018, p. 4). While the CAHME criteria emphasize competency development, they do not identify specific competencies for accreditation and leave it to educational institutions to identify and adopt a competency model. Educational institutions for their part have either adapted some of the major competency models such as National Center for Healthcare Leadership, Healthcare Leadership Alliance, and Saint Louis University. These competency models are broad and overarching and have several domains within which competencies are categorized. Competencies relevant to research methods and analytics would be a subset of domains such as critical thinking, information management, performance management, problem-solving, and communication.

Through competencies there is a clear focus on application–orientation of research methods and analytics courses. This requires the ability to not only understand available data and the methods that can be brought to bear upon them but also be able to apply these in the work environment. In order to do so, familiarity with tools and software that interface with data and ease in using and applying these tools and software is required.

1.2.3 Existing Resources

To address the needs of competency-based education in research methods and analytics, there is a range of texts from the theoretical to the very practical. Two books (Kros & Rosenthal, 2016; Quirk, 2016) that are currently based on Excel and have direct healthcare applications are statistical-based and limit themselves to a quantitative-only approach besides other limitations. This field needs to be enriched through this textbook that expands the quantitative boundary to include text analysis as well as the use of maps through a more comprehensive and current approach with direct application of relevant real-world data from healthcare.

1.3 Outline of the Book

In order to be responsive to the needs of a competency-based, application-oriented,comprehensive, and yet nimble approach to research methods and analytics in a rapidly evolving healthcare environment deluged with data, this book covers select content. The basis of this book is application of Excel to interface with a variety of data (quantitative and qualitative) and apply the extended repertoire of tests and analyses (through Add-ins) in Excel and interpret these tests and analyses for decision-making. Thus, Chapter 2, Working in Excel® and Importing Healthcare Data, provides familiarity with the Excel environment, uses sample data to go through the basic steps in importing data from a variety of formats, and then manages data to get them ready for analysis. The process of including and activating Add-ins in Excel for Analysis ToolPak and 3D Maps as well as installing MeaningCloud is also covered. Next, in Chapter 3, Identifying, Categorizing, and Presenting Healthcare Data Using Excel®, we look at ways in which the level of measurement of our data affects choice of summary and description of data distribution. In this chapter, we consider representing our data through pivot tables and pivot charts as well as several chart types that are available through Excel.

Having covered the importation and initial management and representation of data, we proceed to Chapter 4, Setting Bounds for Healthcare Data and Hypothesis Testing Using Excel®, to use Excel to establish 95% confidence intervals around measures of sample data and then use these bounds for testing hypotheses about the underlying population. These steps lead to undertaking Z-test for testing hypotheses about the population mean and comparing two samples. While in Chapter 5, Testing and Comparing Means of Healthcare Datasets Using Excel®, we use the t-test in Excel to compare the means of two groups of data. Variations of the t-test allow us to make different assumptions about the underlying population.

After our initial foray into analysis and tests in Excel, in Chapter 6, Checking Patterns in Healthcare Data Using Scatterplots, Correlations, and Regressions in Excel®, we use scatter plots, correlations, and regressions in Excel to understand the relationship and patterns in data. In Chapter 7, Visualization and Spatial Analysis of Healthcare Data Using 3D Maps in Excel®, we use 3D Maps in Excel to visualize and analyze data in three dimensions. In addition to three-dimensional maps, this feature within Excel uses time variables in data to also visualize a video of data aggregation.

In Chapter 8, Using Analysis of Variance (ANOVA) in Healthcare Datasets to Compare Groups and Test Hypotheses in Excel®, we use the analysis of variance (ANOVA) test in Excel to compare three or more groups or categories and test hypotheses about their mean values. Having covered the frequently used quantitative analyses in Excel, we proceed in Chapter 9, Text Analysis of Healthcare Data Using MeaningCloud Add-In in Excel®, to use the MeaningCloud Add-In in Excel to perform several types of qualitative analysis. A hypothetical example is used for text classification, sentiment analysis, topic extraction, and text clustering. Finally, in Chapter 10, Sampling and Research Design Using Healthcare Data in Excel®, we go through a brief review of common sampling and research designs. Examples in Excel are used to describe the process of sampling under the different approaches and considerations in hypothesis testing and issues of generalizability from sample to population.

1.4 Competency Development

The content of this book (see earlier section on "Outline of the Book") is selected to provide coverage of competencies in research methods and analytics (see Table 1.2). Five competency domains spanning critical thinking, information management, performance management, problem-solving, and communication are identified for coverage through the content in this book. Based on the emphasis within each of the chapters, competency domains of critical thinking and problem-solving are covered in each of the chapters. The competency domain of information management is emphasized in the chapters pertaining to getting data ready for use and presenting these data in Excel as well as the spatial and text analyses. Through the chapters devoted to quantitative analysis, the competency domain of problem-solving is covered. Finally, the competency domain of communication is covered in the chapters on presenting data in Excel as well as spatial analysis of data.

Clearly, there is an overlap of competency domains within this text. Equally, depending on how this content is used, it is possible to increase or decrease this overlap of competency domains as well as build in coverage of competency domains not identified here.

In Box 1.1, the scenario identified a deluge of data in healthcare from electronic medical records and the interconnectedness of billing and claims together with social determinants of health and surveys from patients

TABLE 1.2 Competency Coverage by Chapter

CHAPTER	COMPETENCY DOMAIN				
	CRITICAL THINKING	INFORMATION MANAGEMENT	PERFORMANCE MANAGEMENT	PROBLEM-SOLVING	COMMUNICATION
2. Working in Excel	✓	✓		✓	
3. Identifying, Categorizing and Presenting Data	✓	✓		✓	✓
4. Bounds and Hypotheses Testing		✓	✓	✓	
5. Testing the Mean	✓	✓	✓	✓	
6. Checking Patterns in Data	✓	✓	✓	✓	
7. Spatial Analysis Using MeaningCloud	✓	✓		✓	✓
8. Analysis of Variance (ANOVA)		✓	✓	✓	
9. Text Analysis	✓	✓		✓	
10. Sampling and Research Design		✓		✓	

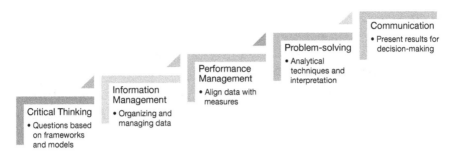

FIGURE 1.2 Application of competency domains.

and providers. There is a need for a sense of purpose in using available data for analysis and decision-making. This sense of purpose is imparted by identifying the problem that needs to be addressed or a question that needs to be answered. These problems and questions can be sourced from guiding frameworks such as the Triple Aim. Frameworks such as these address critical thinking domains (Figure 1.2) to better choose data that would provide the solutions to our problems and questions. Following this important first step, the ability to organize and manage these disparate sources of healthcare data is what the information management domain is all about. This is a critical step because, if there are clutter and disarray in managing data, it will be impossible to use them for analysis and making decisions. Clutter and disarray in data could arise on account of data not being in a usable format. Having data in a usable format would make it amenable to consider what specific measures these data represent. Generating values of these measures would then facilitate the monitoring of progress on these measures and thus address the performance management domain.

Collecting and sifting through data are not an end. These data are to be responsive to specific questions that need answers—our starting point. Here the competency domain of problem-solving aids the use of applicable analytical techniques to compute and interpret the results and provide answers. Finally, the presentation of results of these analyses that informs decision-making addresses the communication domain.

1.5 Summary

In healthcare, there is an increasing number of sources of data such as EHR, Billing, Social Determinants of Health, and surveys of patient experience such as HCAHPS. For these data sources to be better used for decision-making, we rely on frameworks such as the Triple Aim to monitor patient experiences, population health, and per capita costs.

The range of data that is available needs to be managed as part of a comprehensive approach that covers quantitative and qualitative approaches and includes spatial analysis also. Excel, through available Add-ins, lends itself to this comprehensive approach to collect, analyze, visualize, and present data. Used thus, Excel facilitates the development of competency domains of critical thinking, information management, performance management, problem-solving, and communication.

1.6 Discussion Questions

1.6.1 What are the sources of healthcare data that you use? For what do you use these healthcare data?

1.6.2 Consider the past year. Within this year, what kinds of decisions have you made based on healthcare data? In considering your decisions, take on whatever role (client, provider, professional, etc.) you play in the healthcare system.

1.6.3 Critique the comprehensive approach to data and analysis put forth in this chapter.

1.6.4 Thus far, what are the ways that you have used Excel for data and analysis? Do you see a role for Excel in accessing a variety of data and analysis in healthcare? Why or why not?

1.6.5 The content in this book aims to cover five competency domains. Of these competency domains, which do you consider to be the most important and which the least? Why?

References

Bell, P. C., & Zaric, G. (2013). *Analytics for managers: With Excel* (1st ed.). New York, NY: Routledge.

Brown, G. D., Patrick, T. B., & Pasupathy, K. S. (Eds.). (2012). *Health informatics: A systems perspective.* Chicago, IL: Health Administration Press.

Commission on Accreditation of Healthcare Management Education. (2018). *CAHME eligibility requirements.* Retrieved from https://www.cahme.org/files/accreditation/ FALL2017_CAHME_CRITERIA_FOR_ACCREDITATION_2018_06_01.pdf

Institute for Healthcare Improvement. (2012). The IHI Triple Aim. Retrieved from http://www.ihi.org:80/Engage/Initiatives/TripleAim/Pages/default.aspx

Institute of Medicine. (2001). *Crossing the quality chasm: A new health system for the 21st century.* Washington, DC: National Academies Press.

Iosebashvili, I. (2018, October 5). The first rule of Microsoft Excel—Don't tell anyone you're good at It. *Wall Street Journal.* Retrieved from https://www.wsj.com/articles/ the-first-rule-of-microsoft-exceldont-tell-anyone-youre-good-at-it-1538754380

Kros, J. F., & Rosenthal, D. A. (2016). *Statistics for health care management and administration: Working with Excel* (3rd ed.). San Francisco, CA: Jossey-Bass.

Quirk, T. J. (2016). *Excel 2016 for health services management statistics: A guide to solving practical problems.* New York, NY: Springer.

2

WORKING IN EXCEL® AND IMPORTING HEALTHCARE DATA

LEARNING OBJECTIVES

- Access relevant sources of healthcare data
- Classify sources of healthcare data
- Use healthcare data for actionable insights
- Appreciate the proper use of Excel in converting data to actionable insights
- Undertake steps to import a variety of healthcare data files for use in Excel
- Gain familiarity with the Excel workspace for managing data
- Learn to identify and address imperfections in data
- Invoke and activate extended capabilities for analysis and visualization in Excel

In this chapter, we start by describing sources of healthcare data and the decisions that the analysis of data leads to before gaining familiarity with the Excel environment, then using sample data to go through the basic steps in importing data from a variety of formats, and then managing data with imperfections to get it ready for analysis. Add-ins in Excel for Analysis ToolPak and 3D Maps as well as installing MeaningCloud are also covered. In this chapter, the competency domains of critical thinking, information management, and problem-solving are emphasized.

Throughout the chapter supplemental content is available for the datasets and tutorial videos. Video availability is denoted with an icon. To gain access to these items, please visit the following urls:

Datasets: https://connect.springerpub.com/content/book/978-0-8261-5028-8

⊙ Tutorial Videos: https://connect.springerpub.com/content/book/978-0-8261-5028-8/chapter/ch11

Box 2.1 highlights many of the sources of data within healthcare institutions—clinical data, cost data, claims data, patient-generated data, pharmaceutical data, patient preferences, and genomic data (Compton-Phillips, 2017). Going from the specific institutional setting to the general healthcare environment, let us map out several sources of data used in healthcare.

BOX 2.1 HEALTHCARE DATA NOW AND IN THE FUTURE

In January 2017, the New England Journal of Medicine (NEJM) Group at Massachusetts Medical Society sent an online survey to its Catalyst Insight Council to get responses to data at healthcare facilities and its usefulness. Members of this council are drawn from "[e]xecutives, clinical leaders, and clinicians at organizations directly involved with health care delivery" (Compton-Phillips, 2017, p. 13). Based on 682 completed surveys, clinical data, cost data, claims data, patient-generated data, pharmaceutical data, and patient preferences (e.g., Hospital Consumer Assessment of Healthcare Providers and Systems [HCAHPS]) data are ranked in order of usefulness as current key sources of data in healthcare by 20% or more of respondents (see Figure 2.1). Given the rapid pace of change in healthcare data, these respondents consider in five-year time, clinical data, cost data, patient-generated data, genomic data, claims data, and patient preferences ranked in order of usefulness as key sources of data in healthcare by 20% or more of respondents. These changes in usefulness over time are reflected across healthcare executives, clinical leaders, as well as clinicians.

Changes in the ranked usefulness of various sources of data during the 5-year forecast are fueled largely by perceived declines in usefulness of pharmaceutical data, claims data, and clinical data as well as perceived increases in usefulness largely of genomic data and patient-generated data. Sandwiched within these trends is the maturing of personalized medicine and a continued concern with cost data.

In addition to other aspects of healthcare data, the survey includes responses to effectiveness of the use of data as well as biggest opportunities for use of data. Forty percent of respondents are unequivocal in stating that they consider their organization's effectiveness of the use of data for direct patient care as "not very" or "not at all" effective and only 20% considered it to be "very" or "extremely" effective. Eighty percent of respondents chose coordination and decision-support and 68% of respondents chose predictive analytics as their top three opportunities for the use of data in healthcare.

The results of this survey, although limited in scope to data from healthcare facilities, point to the growing importance of sources of data

(continued)

BOX 2.1 (*continued*)

in healthcare and how current efforts to use these data are still a work in progress—a lot still needs to be done. With the changes in importance of sources of data, the ability to manage these data and use them timely for decision-making is highlighted.

Most Useful Sources of Health Care Data Today and in 5 Years

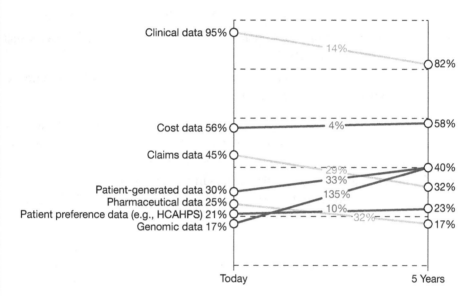

What do you consider the top three most useful sources of health care data today and in 5 years?

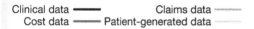

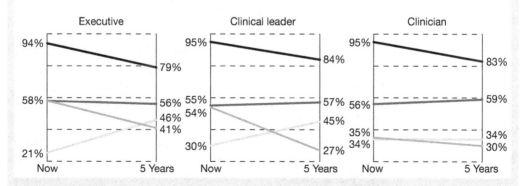

FIGURE 2.1 Changing sources of healthcare data.

NOTE: Base = 682 (Multiple responses).

SOURCE: Compton-Phillips, A. (2017). What data can really do for health care [NEJM Catalyst Insight Report]. Retrieved from http://join.catalyst.nejm.org/hubfs/Insights%20Council%20Monthly%20-%20 Files/Insights%20Council%20March%202017%20Report%20What%20Data%20Can%20Really%20 Do%20for%20Health%20Care.pdf. © Massachusetts Medical Society

2.1 Sources of Healthcare Data

For healthcare, there are several sources of data that students, practitioners, and other decision-makers need to keep abreast of. Broadly classified, these include (National Library of Medicine, n.d.):

a. Population surveys—a rich source of constantly updated social, economic, demographic, health, and other data

b. Survey of providers—periodic surveys of healthcare providers and healthcare institutions

c. Vital statistics—records of births, deaths, and other life events

d. Registry of diseases—periodically updated records of diseases such as cancer and AIDS

e. Administrative records—records compiled based on interaction or stay at a healthcare institution

As a user of healthcare data, a rich repository is accessed through the Agency for Healthcare Research and Quality (AHRQ; www.ahrq.gov/data/resources/index.html). These data sources span population surveys, surveys of providers, and administrative records in our broad classification of sources of data (see Section 2.1). Data that can be accessed pursuant to data use agreements include:

a. Consumer Assessment of Healthcare Providers and Systems (CAHPS®)—In 1995, AHRQ initiated surveys to collect patient experiences from their interactions with healthcare providers and systems. Over the years, this has become more specialized and includes a variety of institutional settings, specific healthcare providers, as well as specific conditions. These administrative records of patient interactions are submitted to AHRQ and facilitate comparison of scores on a variety of CAHPS measures across institutional as well as state and national levels.

b. Healthcare Cost and Utilization Project (HCUP)—In 1988, AHRQ began surveys to collect information on hospital care including inpatient stay, surgical and service visits, and use of the emergency department. This population survey is now considered the most comprehensive source of hospital care data in the United States.

c. Medical Expenditure Panel Survey (MEPS)—In 1996, AHRQ designed large-scale panel (same respondent is surveyed for surveys in later years) surveys of families, individuals, healthcare providers and employers to collect data on cost and use of healthcare, including health insurance coverage. Since these population surveys follow the same individuals, the design of these surveys provides representative samples at national and state levels for inpatient and emergency department visits.

d. Survey on Patient Safety (SOPS) Culture™—In 2004, AHRQ developed and released an SOPS and culture for providers and staff at hospitals. Over the years, this survey of providers and staff for assessing organizational patient safety and culture has expanded beyond hospitals to include medical offices, nursing homes, community pharmacies, and ambulatory surgery centers.

There are several important sources of population survey data. Two sources serve as clearing houses and consolidators of population survey data from a variety of sources. One is exclusively focused on the United States and provides the County Health Rankings (http://www.countyhealthrankings.org/explore-health-rankings/use-data/exploring-data). Since 2010, these rankings and data, including socioeconomic, demographic, health, and environmental topics, are available and updated each year. In its most recent round of data update in 2018, over 20 sources of periodic population surveys and registries conducted by a variety of organizations and agencies were used. Another source of global and domestic data that are sourced from a variety of population surveys and periodically updated is through the Institute for Health Metrics and Evaluation (www.healthdata.org). Initially established in 2007 with funding from The Bill and Melinda Gates Foundation and the state of Washington, the Institute has a close partnership with the University of Washington and provides national and international data on a variety of health subjects and uses models and prediction for the burden of disease estimates (Institute for Health Metrics and Evaluation, n.d.). Both these sources provide a variety of reports as well as tools for visualizing data and downloading data for additional analysis. An additional source, especially suited to students and researchers with access, is the Inter-university Consortium for Political and Social Research's (ICPSR) 272 survey series categorized under healthcare facilities (www.icpsr.umich.edu/icpsrweb/ICPSR/search/studies?CLASSIF_FACET=ICPSR.IX). These surveys are national and international on a variety of socioeconomic, demographic, and health topics and span over 5 million variables.

Key sources of vital statistics (births, deaths, divorce, etc.) and registries (cancer, toxic substances, immunization, other specific conditions, etc.) are at the Centers for Disease Control and Prevention (CDC; www.cdc.gov/nchs/data_access/ftp_data.htm). The public use datasets through these agencies and offices within the CDC are large and use file transfer protocol (ftp) for downloading and using these datasets.

Examples of administrative records that are collected by AHRQ (see Section 2.1) include the CAHPS as well as SOPS Culture. There are other administrative records, especially health insurance claims data. Since these contain sensitive financial information, much of these data are not easily accessible. However, state and regional efforts around compiling All-Payer Claims Database (APCD) were underway and in 2007, there was a greater push to expand the boundaries of this claims database leading to the establishment in 2010 of the APCD Council (n.d.). In addition to these public sources of healthcare data, FairHealth (www.fairhealth.org/data) is a commercial source of private and Medicare claims data.

In this section, we have identified several sources of data. In Chapter 12, List of Select Sources of Healthcare Data, these sources of data are compiled and categorized using the National Library of Medicine's classification referenced earlier in this section. This compilation also includes brief notes on these sources of data as well as websites from which these data are available. However, these data are only as good as the decisions that we make using these data.

2.2 Data Used for Decision-Making

When we are faced with this growing flood from the rapid availability of data, the next fear is the "paralysis of analysis." When you are drowning in data, there is nothing much that you can do other than struggle to just stay afloat and watch helplessly as the data escapes all around you. Rather than be faced with this predicament, let us see what are the ways in which we can harness this data to make decisions from it.

In a time of rapid change in the healthcare environment, the Commission on Accreditation of Healthcare Management Education exhorts academic institutions to prepare healthcare management students with the "analytical, financial, quality improvement, technology, and problem solving skills that will add value immediately to their organizations" (Commission on Accreditation of Healthcare Management Education, 2016, p. 8). These skills facilitate decision-making in a variety of key functional areas and span the continuum of areas in the Triple Aim of improving patient experience, improving population health, and reducing the per capita cost of care (Institute for Healthcare Improvement, 2012).

The push to work smarter with all the data around us is also evident in the several white papers, reports, and articles that are authored by organizations with a business intelligence offering. Organizations such as Google, IBM, and McKinsey and Company all emphasize the continuum of data—insights—action (Dykes, 2016; IBM Analytics, 2015; Mohr & Hurtgen, 2018). This continuum conveys the need to identify, gather, and work with relevant raw data in order to analyze and generate predictive analytics or insights into what the trends are, and then use these insights for prescriptive analytics or actions related to what decisions the organization can take based on these insights.

2.2.1 Actionable Insights

Having identified several sources of data in the previous section, let us see how actionable insights can be drawn from such diverse sources of data. In Figure 2.2, the broad classification of sources of healthcare data is our starting point. These five commonly used categories of data provide rich data on several topics as identified through select examples for each category of data. Lest these data be relegated to just a heap of data points that do not make sense, we need to be able to analyze these data to draw insights and visually display this information. However, we cannot stop and rest on our laurels at this point as the work is incomplete till this insight is made actionable.

- Population surveys, such as longitudinal data within the MEPS, are used to provide insights related to the market and population that is served by a health entity. The insights from such population surveys could also be about health needs assessment for communities that are served by a health entity or even to forecast demand from target populations. Actions based on these insights include being the basis for planning focus areas and/or expansion of services and facilities by a health entity.

- Survey of providers, such as SOPS Culture, is used to provide insights about work performance as well as flag possible workflow issues. Actions based on these insights include specific and targeted quality and performance improvement.

- Data from vital statistics and registries, such as births/deaths and cancer, respectively provide insights about markets and populations served as well as health needs assessment, and they forecast demand from target populations. Actions based on these insights include additional research or analysis to identify root-cause of specific problems flagged through vital statistics or registry data as well as using data from these sources to supplement strategic planning by health entities.

Data	Insights	Action
Population Surveys (e.g. Medical Expenditure Panel Survey (MEPS))	Market research; health needs assessment; forecast of demand	Planning areas for focus and/or expansion;
Survey of Providers (e.g. Survey on Patient Safety (SOP) Culture™)	Performance monitoring; current issues in workflows;	Process and quality improvement
Vital Statistics (e.g. births and deaths – National Center for Health Statistics (NCHS))	Market research; health needs assessment; forecast of demand	Root-cause analysis; supplement to strategic planning
Registry (e.g. cancer registry – Centers for Disease Control and Prevention (CDC))	Market research; health needs assessment; forecast of demand	Root-cause analysis; supplement to strategic planning
Administrative Records (e.g. claims data with organizations and state/national All-Payer Claims Database (APCD))	Performance monitoring; Revenues; comparison to peer institutions	Process and quality improvement; revenue cycle management

FIGURE 2.2 Using healthcare data for decision-making.

■ Administrative records such as claims data with organizations and state and national APCD provide insights about the performance of health entities as well as how their revenues stack up against their competition. Actions based on these insights include targeted process and quality improvements that lead to better revenue cycle management and help health entities to manage their cash flows and liquidity.

This overview of some of the common sources of healthcare data as well as possible insights and actions based on these data shows how data can be a starting point for actions. It is very easy to have numerous data points; however, if these are not analyzed and visualized to draw out insights that can inform actions, data collection will be meaningless. Despite their best intentions, less than a third of organizations are data-driven with the missing piece invariably being actionable insights that can be acted upon (Dykes, 2016).

2.3 Excel in Actionable Insights

Wizardry in the intricacies of Excel is the current rage and a much sought-after status in office circles (Iosebashvili, 2018). This speaks of the tremendous capabilities within this software that are waiting to be tapped to mine insights from data. Over the years and with each successive version, the boundaries are being stretched and new features and Add-ins becoming available in this software. The current version of Excel has 1,048,576 rows and 16,384 columns which translates to over 17 billion cells in which to store data. Given the sheer volume of cells there is a tremendous amount of data that can be readily crunched and analyzed to provide actionable insights. Yes, in the realm of big data this volume of data space in Excel is likely to be exceeded. However, for those exceptional analyses, you are likely to need greater computing power as well as specialized analyses that are not going to be the norm for everyday users of data.

Having broached the idea of possible limitations in the use of Excel for analysis, it is not out of place to also discuss some of the criticism leveled against the use of Excel. IBM recently produced a paper *The Risks of Using Spreadsheets for Statistical Analysis* (IBM Corporation, 2018) to highlight the usefulness of spreadsheets such as Excel, but also pointing out the limits of using Excel. These limits are apparently due to superficial (not detailed) analysis, unreliable results with large datasets, more time required for analysis on account of lack of specialized data preparation features, complexity in creating spreadsheets, and they can be error prone. While the criticism about managing very large datasets and lack of detailed analysis using Excel may be worth pondering; this needs to be put in context. First, this report came out in 2018 when the expanded capabilities within Excel as well as several recent texts on using Excel in healthcare and other industries were being adopted. Second, it is not often that most practitioners and students will deal with such situations. Third, any computer applications (Excel and specialized statistical software included) are only as smart as the human working with them. And for the rare occasions that these opportunities and needs turn up, most certainly the use of specialized and powerful statistical packages is recommended.

Bearing these caveats in mind, let us see how we can become more familiar with some of the features in Excel that will allow us to make the most of working in this software to draw out insights that can inform actions.

2.4 Importing Data Into Excel

The Excel environment is compatible with several formats of data files (Microsoft Office Support, n.d.). Many file formats in which you can save an Excel file are file formats from which you can import data. Of course, the degree of difficulty in importing data from the less common file formats varies. Nonetheless, there are several common file formats in which data are frequently available and can be easily imported into Excel. These common file formats are .xlsx (Excel 2007 and later workbooks), .xls (earlier version of Excel workbooks), .xml (Extensible Markup Language—a text-based database), .json (JavaScript Object Notation—open standard text file format), .tsv (tab separated values), .txt (text or tab delimited file), .csv (comma delimited file), .dbf (database file), and .ods (OpenDocument Spreadsheet). Among these seemingly disparate file formats, the unifying feature is that data fields are separated by using a delimiter such as space, column, tab, text, comma, or something else.

2.4.1 Importing From .txt or .csv File Format Data Files

As indicated on the first page of the chapter, access is provided via the url for Dataset 1 (https://www.countyhealthrankings.org/explore-health-rankings/rankings-data-documentation/national-data-documentation-2010-2017). This is a .txt file based on the 2017 County Health Rankings Data (www.countyhealthrankings.org) that can be imported for use in Excel through the following steps. These steps are common to importing files that are .txt or .csv format.

1. Step 1: Open Excel and navigate to the file location on your computer by using File > Open > Browse. Make sure that the type of file for which you are looking is either "All Files" or ".txt or .csv." Open the .txt file and you will be prompted with the following Dialog Box (Figure 2.3) Text Import Wizard Step 1 of 3. In most cases, this Wizard will correctly identify that your data file is delimited and the kind of delimiter used—in this case tabs.

2. Step 2 of this Wizard, the dialog box (Figure 2.3) will provide you further options to confirm your choice of delimiter as well as a preview of how the choice of delimiter affects the data that you are about to import. In most cases, the delimiter is "tab" and the preview of the

Tutorial video for Sections 2.4.1 and 2.4.2 is available by accessing the following url: https://connect.springerpub.com/content/book/978-0-8261-5028-8/chapter/ch11

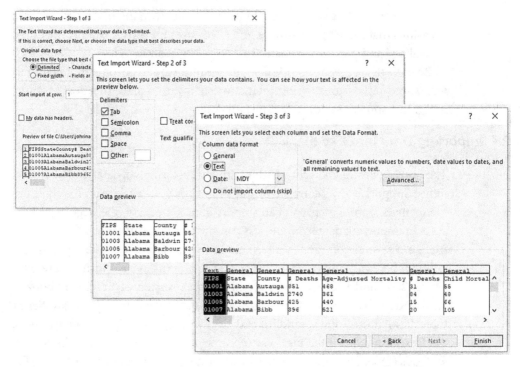

FIGURE 2.3 Importing text file for use in Excel.

data shows that the fields and the data therein appear to be correctly displayed.

3. Step 3 of this Text Import Wizard allows you to fine-tune the kind of data in each of the columns identified through your delimiter (Step 2). In most frequent use of this wizard, you can skip this step by choosing "Finish" (see Figure 2.3). Here, just for the first column "FIPS" we use "text" for the type of data in this column and leave as "general" for all other columns of data. By identifying FIPS as "text" it helps to preserve the initial zero that is used in the code. If we had chosen "general" for the data in the FIPS column, we would have lost the initial zero. Once you complete all steps of the Data Import Wizard, make sure to save your file as an Excel Workbook (.xlsx).

2.4.2 Managing Worksheets

Once you have saved your workbook and before making any changes, it is a good idea to keep data in its original form in case you need to retrieve it. One way to do so is to save your original worksheet with the name "original." Excel contains several worksheets that are identified by tabs at the bottom (Figure 2.4). If you right-click this tab, you have options to rename the worksheet. Go ahead and rename it as "original." Now once again right-click the "original" worksheet tab. One of the options that is available is to "Move

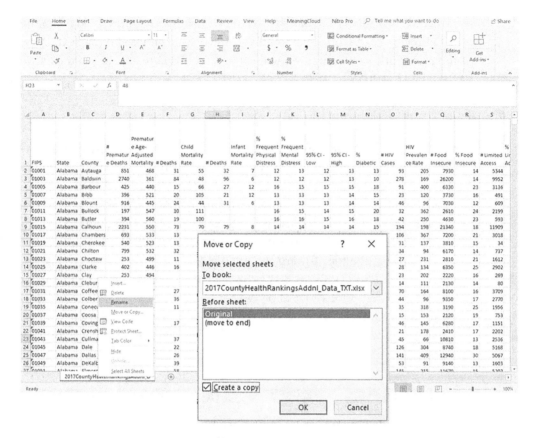

FIGURE 2.4 Managing worksheets.

or Copy." Choose this option and in the tab that opens, go ahead and select "move to end" and check the box against "create copy" (Figure 2.4). As a result of these steps, you have now created a copy "Original 2" of your original worksheet. In order to not get confused, go ahead and rename the worksheet "Original 2" as "copy." Now you can make all your changes in the worksheet "Copy" and not have to fret about losing the original data.

2.5 Editing Cells and Content

2.5.1 Aligning Content in Cells

Notice that the first row contains the field name. In some cells, the field name may not be completely visible. Fix this easily by selecting the row (click on the number "1" on the extreme left-hand side—indicating the first row) and go to "Alignment" on the Tool Ribbon. Click on the down arrow there to

Tutorial video for Sections 2.5.1 and 2.5.2 is available by accessing the following url: https://connect.springerpub.com/content/book/978-0-8261-5028-8/chapter/ch11

reveal the "Format Cells" dialog box. In this dialog box, you should be on the "Alignment" tab. Scroll down to "Text Control" and choose "Wrap Text." Now the row width for the first cell will expand and you are able to see the entire field name within each cell.

2.5.2 Visual Examination of Data

Since this is a large dataset, as a first step, let us undertake a visual examination of the data. A quick and easy way to undertake this is by using the "Freeze Panes" option (Figure 2.5). This option freezes or makes static certain rows, columns, or both. To "Freeze Panes" place your cursor in cell D2 (Column D, Row 2). This is the cell that has FIPS, State, and County columns to the left and the row with headers above it. With the cursor in cell D2, click on "View" in the menu at the top. Toward the middle of the "View" menu options you have "Freeze Panes." Click on the down arrow next to "Freeze Panes" and you have three options that allow you to either freeze both rows and columns, rows above, or columns to the left of the cell currently chosen. Choose the "Freeze Panes" option. Now, the header row and the columns with FIPS,

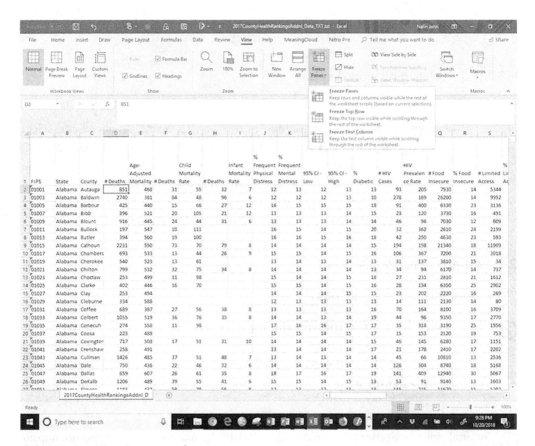

FIGURE 2.5 Viewing your data.

State, and County are fixed and the data in the remaining cells will scroll. The advantage of freezing panes is that it allows you to have a reference point and relate the data to what specifically it refers to since the header rows as well as FIPS, State, and County information can now be easily cross-referenced for each cell with data.

2.6 Managing Data

When data has been imported in Excel, before it can be used, it is important to examine and/or prepare the data for use. In the perfect world, this step would not be required as the data would be complete, clean, and correct. However, in the real world, this situation invariably does not obtain. The reality is that we invariably deal with "muddy data," that is, data are either not complete (missing data on cases and/or variables), not clean (data do not fit into neat columns or rows and columns of data are swapped), or not correct (data do not fit into neat columns or variable fields are non-numeric). Each of these 3C's has the potential to attenuate the usable data resulting in complete records and/or data on certain variables being invalidated for analysis. Faced with such situations, we are likely to not be able to run the analysis or end up running the analysis only on the usable subset of the data. In this section, we explore some of the common issues and how to address them during analysis.

2.6.1 Missing Data

Incomplete data or missing data are the most common occurrences when managing data. Missing data could be on account of missing complete records or missing data on some variables in your dataset. Going back to Figure 2.5, you will notice that there are several blank cells for the various infant and child mortality measures. In the complete data table, data on these measures are missing for several records. In order to determine if missing data is a problem, first we need to determine the extent of this problem. Two approaches to identifying the extent of missing data is through either highlighting blank data cells or counting the number of blank data cells.

    a. Highlight blank data cells—In order to highlight blank data cells, choose the entire column of data. Once this is done, press F5 to access the "Go To" window (Figure 2.6) and click on the "Special" tab at the bottom of this window. In the "Go To Special" window that opens, choose "Blank" and click "OK." Now all the blank cells in this column of data are highlighted and you can go ahead and choose a highlight color to make these blank data cells stand out.

Tutorial video for Section 2.6.1 is available by accessing the following url: https://connect .springerpub.com/content/book/978-0-8261-5028-8/chapter/ch11

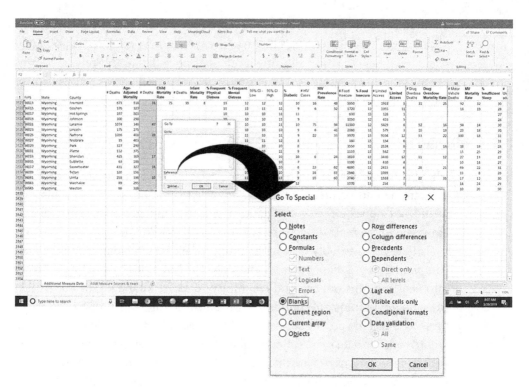

FIGURE 2.6 Highlighting blank data cells.

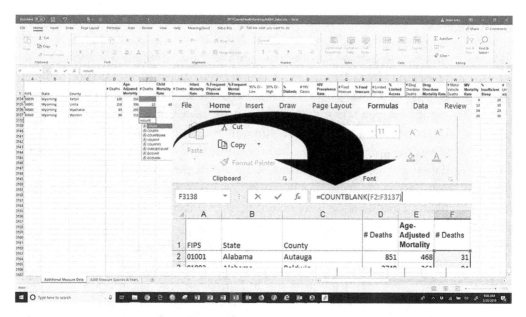

FIGURE 2.7 Counting blank data cells.

b. Counting blank data cells—In order to get a precise count of the number of blank data cells, go to an empty cell in your workbook and type in this empty cell "=COUNTBLANK" (Figure 2.7). In this formula, you are then prompted to select the range of cells for which this count of blank cells is required. Go ahead and select the cells and close the parentheses in the formula before pressing "Enter." In the cell in which this formula for counting the number of blank cells is input, you get a precise count of the number of blank data cells. In this case it is 1,193 out of 3,136 counties that are missing data on the number of child deaths or 38% of counties.

For this large data table on counties, more than one in three counties is missing data on child deaths. This is a large amount of missing data that cannot be ignored and brushed aside for any analysis that includes child deaths. Should there be a need to include this variable in any analysis, it is important to have clear assumptions about the nature of missing data and then determine ways to address this issue of missing data (see later in this section).

If, however, for this large data table, the percentage of missing data for a variable is less than 10%, it may be easier to address the missing data and proceed with the analysis where this missing data is ignored since this would in most cases provide unbiased estimates (Allison, 2001; Papageorgiou, Grant, Takkenberg, & Mokhles, 2018). However, in working with smaller data tables, missing data can lead to several problems such as loss of statistical power, loss of representation, biased estimates, and increased complexity of statistical analysis (Papageorgiou et al., 2018).

Whenever there is greater than 10% of data missing on a variable, it is imperative not to ignore the missing data and explore and understand assumptions about the data that is missing. This is because missing data may or may not affect conclusions (IBM Corporation, n.d.). Classically (Allison, 2001) the assumptions about missing data are classified as:

- Missing Completely at Random (MCAR)—This is the strongest assumption that any variable that is missing cannot depend on any other variable or even on the potential missing value of the variable.
- Missing at Random (MAR)—This is a strong assumption that any missingness depends on assignment (say to treatment or control) but not on the potential missing value.
- Not Missing at Random (NMAR)—This is not a strong assumption as there is no randomness in the missingness of data.

When the assumption about missing data is MCAR or MAR, missingness is considered ignorable and when it is NMAR, it is considered not ignorable. A variety of specialized software can be used to analyze and better understand the assumptions that can be made about the missing data as well as make corrections whenever the assumption of randomness (MCAR or MAR) is met and missingness is ignorable. Statistical software such as XLStat (within Excel), SPSS, Stata, and SAS have inbuilt routines to better understand and address the issue.

2.6.1.1 APPROACHES TO MISSING DATA

Whenever the missingness is small (<10%) and/or the missingness is ignorable, the approaches to missing data broadly include multiple imputation or using maximum likelihood estimators (Allison, 2001; Blackwell, Honaker, & King, 2017; Papageorgiou et al., 2018). These approaches steer clear of the dangers in just replacing missing values with averages. Imputation to replace missing values based on multiple regressions is discussed and an example is covered in Chapter 6, Checking Patterns in Healthcare Data Using Scatterplots, Correlations, and Regressions in Excel®. See in Chapter 6, Section 6.6 on "Revisiting Missing Values." In fact, deletion of the small number of cases (<10%) containing missing data in most cases still leads to unbiased estimation in regression models (Allison, 2001).

Only a brief overview is provided here and the work of other researchers (Allison, 2001; Papageorgiou et al., 2018) is recommended for more details on the topic of missingness. Additionally, if the missing data problem is deep-rooted, it may require working with a statistician.

2.6.2 Swapping Rows and Columns

At times, depending on the source, data may not always be available in clean and neat columns in Excel. An example of this is the Hospital Consumer Assessment of Healthcare Providers and Systems (HCAHPS) survey from the Veterans Administration (VA) available through www.data.medicare.gov. Dataset 2 is an extract from the VA HCAHPS Survey for Allegheny County and provides data on the 11 composite measures reported from these surveys completed by patients from VA medical facilities. As before (see Section 2.5.1, "Aligning Content in Cells"), let us fix the alignment of the header row to better understand this data. Once the alignment of the header is fixed, you can better see the data (Figure 2.8). Notice that columns J, K, and L show specific questions and responses in rows. For each county with a VA Hospital, the data follows this format and appears in 11 rows—one for each composite measure. To show how this data from rows can be transposed into columns, we focus on just one county.

Start by inserting 11 columns to the right of column L. Next, copy the "Answer Description" in column K (rows 2–12). After copying, place your cursor in the empty cell M1—the first of the 11 columns that you just inserted. Right click to reveal "Paste Options." Choose the fourth option—transpose. This will paste the column that you just chose in the row starting with cell M1. Repeat this process of transposing for the data in column L (L2–L12) and pasting it in M2. Once you have verified that the data from columns K and L have been transposed into rows 1 and 2, go ahead and delete columns J, K, and

Tutorial video for Section 2.6.2 is available by accessing the following url: https://connect .springerpub.com/content/book/978-0-8261-5028-8/chapter/ch11

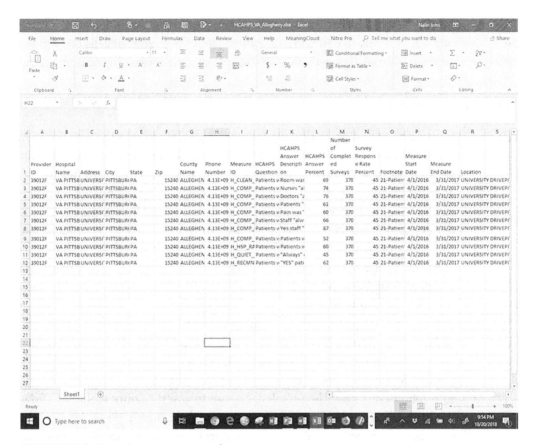

FIGURE 2.8 Data in rows, *not* columns.

L. Next, delete rows 3 to 12. Through these steps, data that were earlier in rows are transposed into the columns and make it easier to analyze within Excel.

2.6.3 Field Types

Continuing with the use of the just modified Dataset 2 where the data was transposed from rows into columns, notice that the column labeled "phone number" shows data under it as "4.13E+09." This is because the number in this cell is currently formatted as scientific notation with E+09 indicating that the decimal place should be moved nine places to the right to get the underlying number without scientific notation. Likewise, E-07 denotes scientific notation where the decimal place must be moved seven places to the left to get the underlying number. Go ahead and right-click the cell with this number. There are several options that open. Toward the bottom, there is the option to "Format Cell." Click on this option and you have a new menu whose tabs reveal various formatting options that can be applied to the cell. The first one is "Number." Click on "Number" and you will see 12 different options to format numbers. Choose "General" and click "OK." The underlying number without scientific notation is now displayed. We undertook this step for just one cell. It is possible to undertake these steps for a range of cells or even the entire workbook if you would like to apply specific formatting of numbers.

2.6.4 Splitting Fields

In working with data, at times it becomes necessary to split the data within a field. The variable in the data field may not be correct as it may be alphanumeric or have additional characters or entry that make the field not usable. Take for example Dataset 3. This file was created using the process of transposing data from rows to columns described earlier. Undertaking this process for all VA facilities in this file and cleaning up results in this file. Notice when you open this file, the first column "Provider ID" contains alphanumeric data. The data in this column consists of six spaces—the first five of which are numbers and the last is the letter "F." We can remove the "F" such that the data in this field is all numeric and can then be better analyzed. To do this, we split this column into a number column and a text column (Winston, 2004). To get started, let us first insert a blank column in-between "Provider ID" and "Hospital Name." Right-click in cell B1 (Hospital Name). From the options revealed, choose "Insert"—it appears just above "Delete." From the sub-options that are now revealed, choose to insert "Entire Column." Now, click on cell A2—the first cell with data in the column "Provider ID." On your keyboard, while holding down "control" and "shift" together, press the "down arrow" key. This step is an easy way to select all the cells with data in the "Provider ID" column. On the menu options above the toolbar, find "Data" and click on it. From the options that are revealed, toward the middle is the option "Text to Columns." Choosing "Text to Columns" opens a dialog box containing a wizard that guides you through the three steps to split the "Provider ID" field (see Figure 2.9).

1. Step 1: Since our data field does not have any separators, we choose "Fixed Width." In case data in the chosen field is separated by spaces, tabs, or other delimiters, we would have chosen the "Delimited" option. Click "Next."

2. Step 2: Since we have chosen "Fixed Width" in step 1, here we are presented with the option of identifying the fixed point that is to be used to split the field. Notice that you are presented with a data preview with sample data from the chosen column "Provider ID" and a scale just above it. Use your mouse to click on the scale in-between the numeric and alphabet part of the data. This mouse click inserts a line in the data separating the numeric and alphabet part of the data. Click "Next."

Tutorial video for Section 2.6.4 is available by accessing the following url: https://connect.springerpub.com/content/book/978-0-8261-5028-8/chapter/ch11

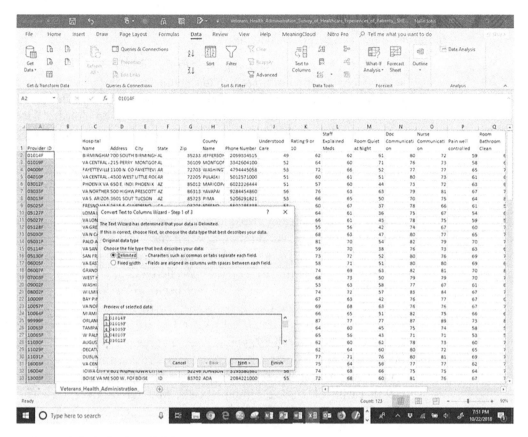

FIGURE 2.9 Splitting fields.

3. Step 3: In this final step, you have the option to choose the type of data in the two fields. For now, we keep the default "general" data type. Click "Finish."

Undertaking these three steps results in the data in the column "Provider ID" splitting into two columns—the updated first column now has only numeric data and the second column now contains the alphabet part of the data. Variations of these basic steps can be used to split data in one column into distinct parts that are more amenable to analysis.

2.6.5 Combining Fields

Another way to correct the data for a variable at times requires combining two or more variable fields. In Excel, just as there are procedures to help spilt a field (column) into two fields (columns), it is also possible to combine two

---

Tutorial video for Section 2.6.5 is available by accessing the following url: https://connect
.springerpub.com/content/book/978-0-8261-5028-8/chapter/ch11

or more fields (columns) into one field (column). There are two ways in which combining fields can be done (Winston, 2004).

1. Using "&" (Ampersand): Going back to the file on HCAHPS Scores with which we were working and had split the Provider ID into numeric and alphabet fields. Now we combine the numeric and alphabet fields. First, insert a column to the right of the newly created alphabet field (in previous step where the Provider ID field was split) and label it "& Combine." In cell C2 in this newly created column, type in the formula =A2&""&B2 and press "Enter" (Figure 2.10). In Excel, all formulae begin with "=" and you can either type in the cell references A2 and B2 in this formula or select the respective cells. The ampersand (&) in the formula is punctuated by two quotation marks. Since there is no space between the two quotation marks, when the two cells are combined there will be no space inserted between the contents of the two cells that are combined. In case a space is needed—as in combining fields "First Name" and "Last Name," all that needs to be done is to ensure that the two quotation marks between the two ampersands include a space. Once you press "Enter," cells A2 and B2 are combined and appear in cell C2. Click on cell C2; you will see that the cell is selected with a border and at the lower right of this cell there is a small square. Use your mouse to drag this square down the column to cell C124—the last cell that will contain the combined cells. Now release the mouse and the cells in column "& Combine" contain the contents of cells A and B.

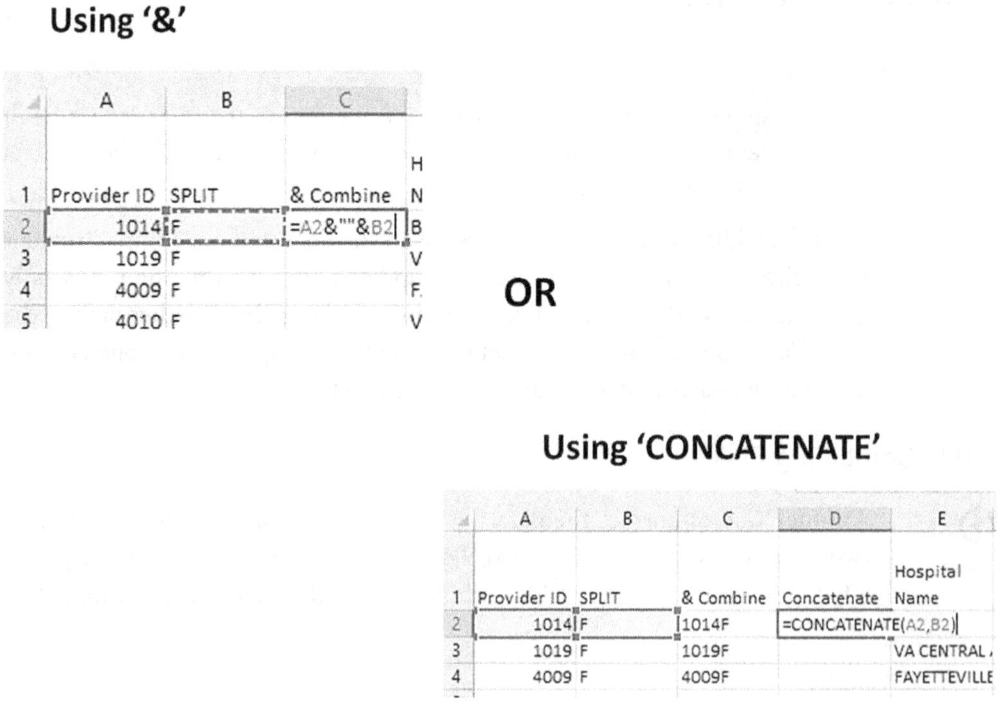

Using '&'

OR

Using 'CONCATENATE'

FIGURE 2.10 Combining fields.

2. Using the function "CONCATENATE": Continuing with the same example just used, the function "Concatenate" is an alternate way to combine two or more fields into one column. First, insert a column before Hospital Name and label it "Concatenate." Next, in cell D2 (in the newly created column), type in the formula =CONCATENATE(A2,B2) and press "Enter" (Figure 2.10). As with using "&", the contents of cells A2 and B2 are now combined. If you click in cell D2 that contains the results of applying this formula, the cell is selected with a square at the bottom right. As before, drag this square down the column to the last row that will contain the combined cell. Note that the Concatenate function is very versatile. In case you need to insert a space between the contents of the cells being combined, the formula would be modified as =CONCATENATE(A2, " ", B2). The space between the quotation marks inserts a space between the contents of cells A2 and B2. It is possible to also merge the contents of the cell A2 and a term such as VA MED CTR. Go ahead and insert an additional column before "Hospital Name." Label this newly created column "Concatenate Character." In cell E2 in this newly created column, type the formula =CONCATENATE(A2, " ", "VA", " ", "CTR"). This formula includes the content of cell A2. Next, the quotation marks with the space inserts a space after the content of cell A2 followed by another space (the next quotation mark with space) and then inserts CTR in cell A2. The result is "1014 VA CTR" in cell E2. As before, go ahead and select cell E2 and drag the small square on the lower right of the selection all the way down to the last row where the content of the combined fields needs to be displayed.

2.7 Managing Add-Ins in Excel

2.7.1 Analysis ToolPak

Certain functionality in Excel is inbuilt but is not activated. A versatile Analysis ToolPak is part of Excel. In order to activate this ToolPak from a worksheet in Excel, click on "File" in the toolbar and scroll down to "Options." Selecting "Options" opens a new panel (Figure 2.11). At the bottom of this panel is "Manage" and "Excel Add-ins" next to it. Click on "Go" which leads to a mini panel (Figure 2.12) with some choices to make. In this mini panel, check the boxes for "Analysis ToolPak" and "Analysis ToolPak—VBA" and click "OK."

Next, repeat the steps to go into "Options" (Figure 2.11), and now when you navigate to "Manage," click on the "down arrow" next to "Excel Add-ins" and select "COM Add-ins"; and click on "Go." In the mini panel that opens (Figure 2.12), make sure to check the box next to "Microsoft Power Map for Excel."

Tutorial video for Section 2.7 is available by accessing the following url: https://connect .springerpub.com/content/book/978-0-8261-5028-8/chapter/ch11

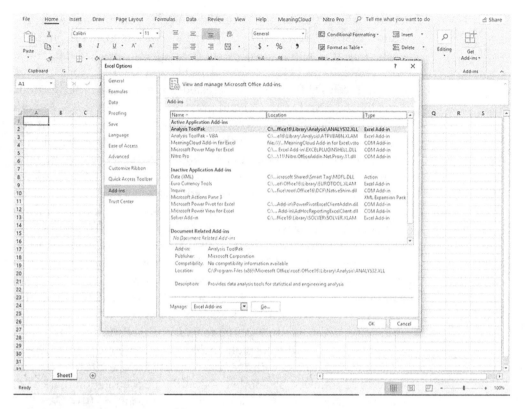

FIGURE 2.11 Managing Add-ins.

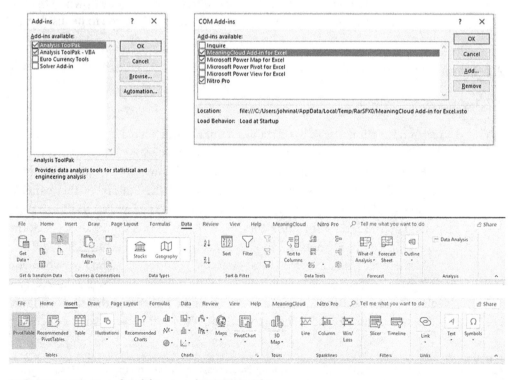

FIGURE 2.12 Excel Add-ins and COM Add-ins.

Having invoked these options, you will likely not notice anything different in Excel. However, if from a worksheet you click on "Data" in the toolbar, the ribbon for "Data" should show a new icon "Data Analysis" as part of the "Analysis" group all the way to the right of your screen. Next, if you click on "Insert" in the toolbar, toward the middle of the ribbon as part of the "Tours" group, you should see an icon "3D Maps." This is different from "Maps" that are part of the "Charts" group in the same ribbon. These icons are your gateway to undertaking several statistical functions and processes in Excel that we explore in this book.

2.7.2 MeaningCloud

Another Add-in that is not in Excel but is available as a free download is the MeaningCloud Add-in (www.meaningcloud.com). Follow the instructions for downloading the Excel Add-in for MeaningCloud and it will then appear in your toolbar in Excel (Figure 2.12). The MeaningCloud Add-in is a useful tool for undertaking text analysis. In Chapter 9, Text Analysis of Healthcare Data Using MeaningCloud Add-In in Excel®, we cover text analysis using this MeaningCloud Add-in.

2.8 Competency Development

Gaining familiarity with working in Excel, including importing and managing data from a variety of formats, is an important information management competency. Box 2.1 underscores this importance by surveying healthcare professionals on sources of healthcare data and their changing usefulness currently and in the future. This survey also brought out our continuing inability to realize the full potential of these data. A critical element of the information management competency domain is the ability to access relevant sources of healthcare data. With the growing availability of data in healthcare spanning population surveys, surveys of providers, vital statistics, registry of diseases, or administrative records—being smart about what data is needed for a specific issue is important in selecting your source of data. This chapter highlights many of the important sources of healthcare data, and Chapter 12, List of Select Sources of Healthcare Data, includes a more comprehensive and categorized listing of sources of healthcare data.

Having identified data for use, this data then needs to be accessed and made available in a useable format in order to make decisions or actionable insights. Specific decisions based on identified sources of data are made using frameworks or models. Making these decisions both about sources of data as well as what to do with the data is what the competency domain of critical thinking is all about. Working with the data to ensure that, regardless of the bewildering array of data formats, they are properly imported for use in Excel; the subsequent work of ironing out issues with variable formats; and cleaning the dataset, including resolving any missing data issues, further strengthens the information management and problem-solving competency domains.

Lastly, by involving the additional capabilities in Excel through managing add-ins such as Analysis ToolPak, 3D-Maps, and MeaningCloud, we can take advantage of more of the functionality in Excel and enhance our information management competency domain.

In this chapter, thinking through and accessing relevant sources and categories of healthcare data provide application of skills centered in the domain of information management. The appropriate use of these data for decision-making focused on Triple Aim or other frameworks, and gaining familiarity with the Excel environment as well as becoming adept at working in this environment is useful for application of skills spanning critical thinking and information management domains. Finally, by managing real-world data with all its imperfections aids skill development and application of both information management as well as problem-solving domains.

2.9 Summary

Healthcare data can be sourced from a variety of governmental, nongovernmental, and commercial entities providing a range of population surveys, surveys with providers, vital statistics, registry of diseases, and administrative records. These data are needed for actionable insights including addressing Triple Aim. However, in order to better use healthcare data, familiarity with the interface in Excel is a good starting point. In gaining this familiarity, it is important to recognize the limitations in using Excel with very large datasets or for very specialized analyses.

In using Excel as the interface, we can import healthcare data in a variety of formats. Prior to using data, checks to ascertain that the data are complete, clean, and correct need to be performed lest data impact the results and interpretation of data. When less than 10% of data is missing at random, the missingness is ignorable and deleting missing records still provides unbiased estimates. In other cases, it is recommended to use specialized software and statistical help to understand the nature of missingness and remediation. Lastly, it is important to invoke some of the latent capabilities and add-ins in Excel to make the most of this versatile software.

2.10 Discussion Questions

2.10.1 This chapter categorizes healthcare data into five categories. Which of these five categories do you consider the most important and which the least? Why?

2.10.2 This chapter categorizes healthcare data into five categories. Which of these five categories is the easiest to access and which the most difficult? Why?

2.10.3 Do you see a role for Excel in converting healthcare data into actionable insights? Why or why not?

2.10.4 If you find that healthcare data with which you are working has many variables that are missing values, how would you approach the use of this data?

2.10.5 If you find that healthcare data has a few missing values, what would you do to address these missing values?

2.11 Practice Problems

All datasets required for the practice problems are available for download at: https://connect.springerpub.com/content/book/978-0-8261-5028-8

2.11.1 You are trying to access a list of counties and county-level sociodemographic data. Unfortunately, the file that you have, Dataset 4, is a text file. Go ahead and import this file into Excel. Once you have the file in Excel, make sure that the data columns line up.

2.11.2 You are an analyst working with a health advocacy group. Your Team Lead has just received a large dataset (Dataset 5) that needs to be analyzed. Your Team Lead alerts you that the data are in a difficult .csv format and he and others in the team have been struggling to get into the data.

    I.   Go ahead and import this file into Excel and save it as an Excel Workbook.

    II.   Lest anybody make changes to the data that are irreversible, go ahead and create a copy of the original worksheet and label them as "Original" and "Copy."

    III.   When you work, make sure to work only in the "Copy" worksheet.

        a.   Go ahead and align cell content such that the entire content in cells is visible and not overlapping.

        b.   Make sure that the state and county codes are formatted as numbers.

        c.   You notice that the county name has "county" after the county name. Go ahead and delete "county" from county name by using split field.

        d.   Combine the state and county codes.

2.11.3 In working at the Veterans Administration you have access to the data in Dataset 3. In this file, the Provider ID is alphanumeric and will not be easily analyzed. Make changes to this column such that it is all numeric.

Tutorial videos provided for Practice Problems 2.11.1–2.11.5 can be accessed by the following url: https://connect.springerpub.com/content/book/978-0-8261-5028-8/chapter/ch11

2.11.4 Your office has been grappling with the worksheet Dataset 6. In a team meeting, the issue is identified as swapping rows and columns. One of the assistants offers to retype the sheet such that the rows and columns are swapped. You suggest that there is an easier way to accomplish this. Go ahead and swap the rows and columns such that years are in rows.

2.11.5 You are undertaking an analysis of child and infant deaths in Alabama using Dataset 7. For this data, a visual examination reveals that there are several missing values for child and infant deaths. In the file, go ahead and highlight and count these missing values.

2.11.6 As the chief data analyst for your hospital, you have been approached by senior management. They have returned from a recent conference where there was renewed buzz around the Triple Aim framework. Smitten by the "Triple Aim" bug, senior management now wants to take the first steps at addressing this framework through concrete data. They reach out to you to identify sources of healthcare data that can address all three aims in the Triple Aim. Use Chapter 12, List of Select Sources of Healthcare Data, or data sources with which you are already familiar, to identify possible sources of data for the Triple Aim.

2.11.7 A health policy think-tank is exploring ways to make sense of the dynamic healthcare landscape. As part of this exploration, the discussion turns to the kinds of data that would help to make sense of this landscape. Rather than leave it to chance that they have addressed the different facets of healthcare, propose a framework (other than the Triple Aim) and identify sources of healthcare data that would provide a multifaceted picture of the dynamic healthcare landscape.

See Chapter 11, Video Tutorials and Answers to Practice Problems Using Healthcare Datasets in Excel®, for video answers to the practice problems.

References

All-Payer Claims Database Council. (n.d.). About APCD Council. Retrieved from https://www.apcdcouncil.org/about-apcd-council

Allison, P. D. (2001). *Missing data* (Vol. 07–136). Thousand Oaks, CA: Sage.

Blackwell, M., Honaker, J., & King, G. (2017). A unified approach to measurement error and missing data: Overview and applications. *Sociological Methods & Research*, 46(3), 303–341. doi:10.1177/0049124115585360

Commission on Accreditation of Healthcare Management Education. (2016). *To be the change: Preparing the future leaders of healthcare*. Retrieved from https://cahme.org/files/Final_CAHME_To_Be_the_Change.pdf

Compton-Phillips, A. (2017). *What data can really do for health care* [NEJM Catalyst Insight Report]. Retrieved from http://join.catalyst.nejm.org/hubfs/Insights%20

Council%20Monthly%20-%20Files/Insights%20Council%20March%202017%20 Report%20What%20Data%20Can%20Really%20Do%20for%20Health%20Care. pdf

Dykes, B. (2016, April 26). Actionable insights: The missing link between data and business value. Retrieved from https://www.forbes.com/sites/brentdykes/2016/04/26/ actionable-insights-the-missing-link-between-data-and-business-value

IBM Analytics. (2015). *From business insight to business action: Combining the power of IBM predictive analytics and IBM decision optimization.* White Paper. Portsmouth, England: IBM Corporation.

IBM Corporation. (2018). *The risks of using spreadsheets for statistical analysis.* Armonk, NY: IBM Corporation. Retrieved from https://www.ibm.com/downloads/ cas/7YEX9BKK

IBM Corporation. (n.d.). IBM SPSS missing values—Overview—United States. Retrieved from https://www.ibm.com/us-en/marketplace/spss-missing-values

Institute for Healthcare Improvement. (2012). The IHI Triple Aim. Retrieved from http://www.ihi.org:80/Engage/Initiatives/TripleAim/Pages/default.aspx

Institute for Health Metrics and Evaluation. (n.d.). History. Retrieved from http:// www.healthdata.org/about/history

Iosebashvili, I. (2018, October 5). The first rule of Microsoft Excel—Don't tell anyone you're good at it. *Wall Street Journal.* Retrieved from https://www.wsj.com/articles/ the-first-rule-of-microsoft-exceldont-tell-anyone-youre-good-at-it-1538754380

Microsoft Office Support. (n.d.). Excel specifications and limits. Retrieved from https://support.office.com/en-us/article/excel-specifications-and-limits- 1672b34d-7043-467e-8e27-269d656771c3

Mohr, N., & Hurtgen, H. (2018, April). *Achieving business impact with data: A comprehensive perspective on the insights value chain* (Report). Dusseldorf, Germany: McKinsey & Co.

National Library of Medicine. (n.d.). Sources of health statistics [Training Material and Manuals]. Retrieved from https://www.nlm.nih.gov/nichsr/usestats/sources. html

Papageorgiou, G., Grant, S. W., Takkenberg, J. J. M., & Mokhles, M. M. (2018). Statistical primer: How to deal with missing data in scientific research? *Interactive CardioVascular and Thoracic Surgery, 27*(2), 153–158. doi:10.1093/icvts/ivy102

Winston, W. L. (2004). *Microsoft Excel: Data analysis and business modeling.* Redmond, WA: Microsoft Press.

3

IDENTIFYING, CATEGORIZING, AND PRESENTING HEALTHCARE DATA USING EXCEL®

LEARNING OBJECTIVES

- Develop questions based on healthcare decision-making
- Use questions to guide selection of data for graphs and charts
- Appreciate the use of level of measurement of data to inform summary of data
- Choose data display through key considerations and questions

In this chapter, the broad theme is to summarize the data. To do this, we are guided by the question that we wish to answer and look at ways in which the level of measurement of data affects choice of summary of data distribution. Next, we consider pivot tables and pivot charts as well as several chart types that are available through Excel. Competencies emphasized in this chapter are critical thinking, information management, problem-solving, and communication.

3.1 Getting Started

Hans Rosling caught the world's attention through his ease with working with global data to effortlessly bring them to life and at the same time convey key messages in the data. His work is found at Gapminder (www.gapminder.org)—an organization that he cofounded to promote "factfulness"—the relaxing

Throughout the chapter supplemental content is available for the dataset and tutorial videos. Video availability is denoted with an icon. To gain access to these items, please visit the following urls:

Datasets: https://connect.springerpub.com/content/book/978-0-8261-5028-8

⊙ Tutorial Videos: https://connect.springerpub.com/content/book/978-0-8261-5028-8/chapter/ch11

habit of carrying opinions that are based on solid facts (and reliable data). Gapminder continues this work by crunching vast amounts of global data to develop visualizations—graphs and figures that are used to tell the story behind the raw numbers. Transforming data into appropriate figures and charts is art with purpose—it starts with a question that needs to be answered.

Having identified several sources and categories of healthcare data as well as decisions that can be made based on those data, we have made a beginning (see Chapter 2, Working in Excel® and Importing Healthcare Data). The decisions that need to be made come from the questions for which we use our data to provide answers. In Box 3.1, transforming 1,990 rows of data into the dashboard with charts and figures is done purposively—identify time trends and geographical distribution together with the top 10 leading causes of death in the United States. Having data for the period 1999–2016, there are several permutations and combinations of data that can be presented. Rather than just a data dump—putting all 1,990 rows of data into a chart—starting with

BOX 3.1 A PICTURE IS WORTH A THOUSAND WORDS

The National Center for Health Statistics (NCHS) within the Centers for Disease Control and Prevention (CDC) is a rich repository of vital statistics—births, deaths, and mortality. In accessing the state level by gender-compressed mortality data files for 1999–2016 from their website (www. cdc.gov/nchs/data_access/cmf.htm), we have 1,990 lines of data. When working with large amounts of data, it is very easy to miss the woods for the trees as the individual data points obfuscate any discernible pattern or relationship that the data might convey. Picture this data table that you can scroll through meaninglessly. From an information standpoint, for policy planners at the national and state levels as well as a variety of stakeholders in healthcare, this is potentially useful information on the healthcare environment, albeit not in its current form. It has data on past trends in mortality that can be the basis for further analysis of causes of mortality as well as finetuning this for geographical locations that may have a preponderance of mortality or steadily declining mortality.

"A picture is worth a thousand words" is a popular idiom that conveys our predicament with this surfeit of data points. If we can convert this data into focused charts and tables that aid discernment of underlying patterns, it will magically transform this data into usable information. On the NCHS website, they have used this and additional data to provide a dynamic dashboard (Figure 3.1). In this figure, the downward trend in mortality rates is evident in the top right panel of this figure (Figure 3.1B), while a map points out the geographical distribution of mortality rates for 2016 (Figure 3.1C). This information is juxtaposed with the top 10 leading causes of death in the United States for 2016 (Figure 3.1A).

(continued)

BOX 3.1 (*continued*)

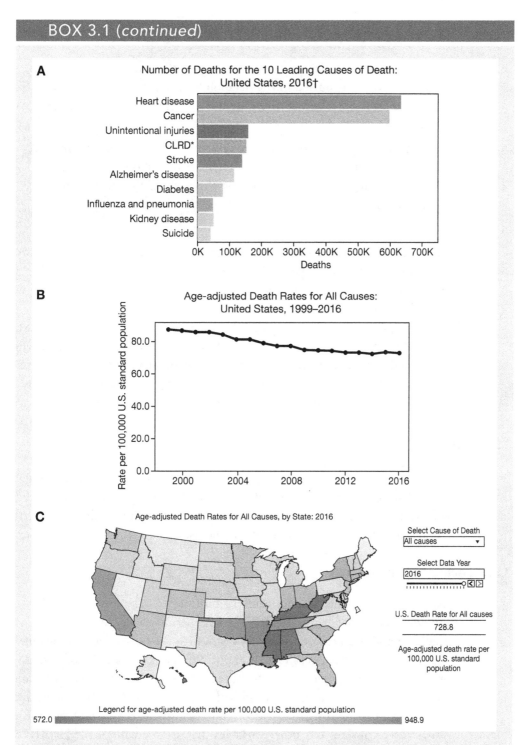

FIGURE 3.1 Leading causes of mortality in the United States, 1999–2017.

SOURCE: Tejada-Vera, B. (2019). Leading causes of death: United States, 1999–2017. National Center for Health Statistics. Retrieved from https://www.cdc.gov/nchs/data-visualization/mortality-leading-causes/index_2.htm

(*continued*)

BOX 3.1 (continued)

Moving from 1,990 rows of data to Figure 3.1 instantly conveyed the message that was buried in the datapoints. The resulting picture, even at a glance, conveys information to policy planners and stakeholders in healthcare.

The transformation of data from raw numbers to focused figures and graphs is a thoughtful process. Starting with a question, you then access and filter data to focus on depicting this information in a form that answers the question.

a question leads to compelling figures. In a White Paper on Visualization, the team at Tableau rightly puts it as: "it is vital that your visualization has a purpose and you are selective about what you include in your visualization to fulfill that purpose" (Tableau, n.d., p. 4).

Starting with a question to guide the purpose is a good beginning. Next, it is important to have some understanding of your data elements that will further aid the identification of specific figures that are better suited to presenting the data. The next section continues the exploration of data elements as a precursor to identifying specific figures later in this chapter.

3.2 Identifying Your Data

Having done the heavy lifting associated with importing data and managing it in Excel, we are now ready to look at ways in which this data can be summarized and presented in preparation for analysis. Our choice of methods and presentation is driven by the level of measurement associated with different variables.

3.2.1 Level of Measurement

In Dataset 3, our dataset on Hospital Consumer Assessment of Healthcare Providers and Systems (HCAHPS) survey at VA facilities (Centers for Medicare and Medicaid Services [CMS], 2016), variables such as Hospital Name, City, County, State, Zip, and Phone Number are examples of nominal or categorical data (Figure 3.2) where the name or number used for inputting data helps us only to categorize or identify different data for our variable but has no other measurement use (Keller, 2006; Schutt, 2015; Singleton & Straits, 2010). If we consider our other variables that are the core of the HCAHPS survey such as Understood Care, rating of 9 or 10, Room Quiet at Night, and so on, these are recorded as percentages and are at interval/ratio level of measurement. At interval/ratio level of measurement, because of fixed intervals (in percentages) we can discuss how far apart two values are or even how many times one value is that of another value. For example, 60% is 40 percentage points away from 20% and 60% is also three times 20%.

Another level of measurement that is not there in the current dataset is the ordinal or rank level of measurement. For the overall HCAHPS survey, this level of measurement appears in the percentile-based star rating of the different components of this survey. Converting these percentages to star ratings makes the measurement level of the variable as ordinal. Thus, since there are not fixed intervals between the star ratings, we can say only that four stars are higher than two stars but not four stars are two times a two stars rating.

The level of measurement of variable needs to be considered as we look at summarizing distributions of these variables. For instance, for variables at nominal or ordinal level of measurement, frequency and percent distributions are appropriate, while for interval and ratio level measurement, a variety of tables, charts, and statistics are possible (Singleton & Straits, 2010).

Provider ID	Hospital Name	Address	City	State	Zip	County Name	Phone Number	Understood Care	Rating 9 or 10	Staff Explained Meds	Room Quiet at Night	Doc Communicati on	Nurse Comm on
01014F	BIRMINGHAM VA MEDICAL CENTER	700 SOUTH 19TH	BIRMINGHAM	AL	35233	JEFFERSON	2059334515	49	62	62	61	80	
01019F	VA CENTRAL ALABAMA HEALTHCARE	215 PERRY HILL RC	MONTGOMERY	AL	36109	MONTGOMERY	3342604100	52	64	60	71	76	
04009F	FAYETTEVILLE AR VA MEDICAL CENTE	1100 N. COLLEGE	FAYETTEVILLE	AR	72703	WASHINGTON	4794445058	53	72	66	52	77	
04010F	VA CENTRAL AR. VETERANS HEALTHC	4300 WEST SEVEN	LITTLE ROCK	AR	72205	PULASKI	5012571000	51	60	61	51	80	
03012F	PHOENIX VA MEDICAL CENTER	650 E. INDIAN SCH	PHOENIX	AZ	85012	MARICOPA	6022226444	51	57	60	44	73	
03033F	VA NORTHERN ARIZONA HEALTHCARE	500 HIGHWAY 89	PRESCOTT	AZ	86313	YAVAPAI	9284454860	56	76	63	63	79	
03013F	VA S. ARIZONA HEALTHCARE SYSTEM	3601 SOUTH SIXTH	TUCSON	AZ	85723	PIMA	5206291821	53	66	65	50	70	
05025F	FRESNO VA MEDICAL CENTER (VA CE	2615 E. CLINTON /	FRESNO	CA	93703	FRESNO	5592285338	53	60	67	37	78	
05127F	LOMA LINDA VA MEDICAL CENTER	11201 BENTON ST	LOMA LINDA	CA	92357	SAN BERNARDI?	9098257084	51	64	61	36	75	
05027F	VA LONG BEACH HEALTHCARE SYSTE	5901 E. SEVENTH	LONG BEACH	CA	90822	LOS ANGELES	5628268000	52	66	61	43	78	
05128F	VA GREATER LOS ANGELES HEALTHCA	11301 WILSHIRE	LOS ANGELES	CA	90073	LOS ANGELES	3104783711	48	55	56	42	74	
05030F	VA N CALIFORNIA HEALTHCARE SYST	10535 HOSPITAL	MATHER	CA	95655	SACRAMENTO	8003828387	52	68	63	47	80	
05031F	PALO ALTO VA MEDICAL CENTER	3801 MIRANDA A	PALO ALTO	CA	94304	SANTA CLARA	6508583939	65	81	70	54	82	
05114F	VA SAN DIEGO HEALTHCARE SYSTEM	3350 LA JOLLA VIL	SAN DIEGO	CA	92161	SAN DIEGO	8585528585	54	59	70	38	76	
05130F	SAN FRANCISCO VA MEDICAL CENTE	4150 CLEMENT ST	SAN FRANCISCO	CA	94121	SAN FRANCISC?	4152214810	54	73	72	52	80	
06005F	VA EASTERN COLORADO HEALTHCAR	1055 CLERMONT	DENVER	CO	80220	DENVER	3033932800	53	58	71	51	80	
06007F	GRAND JUNCTION VA MEDICAL CENT	2121 N. AVENUE	GRAND JUNCTION	CO	81501	MESA	9702441329	61	74	69	63	82	
07003F	WEST HAVEN VA MEDICAL CENTER	950 CAMPBELL AV	WEST HAVEN	CT	6516	NEW HAVEN	2039325711	58	68	73	50	79	
09002F	WASHINGTON DC VA MEDICAL CENT	50 IRVING STREET	WASHINGTON	DC	20422	DISTRICT OF CC	2027458000	49	53	63	58	77	
08002F	WILMINGTON VA MEDICAL CENTER	1601 KIRKWOOD	WILMINGTON	DE	19805	NEW CASTLE	3029942511	64	74	72	57	83	
10009F	BAY PINES VA MEDICAL CENTER	10000 BAY PINES	BAY PINES	FL	33744	PINELLAS	7273986661	55	67	63	42	76	
10057F	VA NORTH FLORIDA/SOUTH GEORG	1601 S W ARCHER	GAINESVILLE	FL	32608	ALACHUA	3523761611	56	69	68	63	76	
10064F	MIAMI VA MEDICAL CENTER	1201 N W 16TH ST	MIAMI	FL	33125	MIAMI-DADE	3053244455	57	66	65	51	82	
99999F	ORLANDO VA MEDICAL CENTER	13800 VETERANS	ORLANDO	FL	32827	ORANGE	4076311000	67	87	77	77	87	
10063F	TAMPA VA MEDICAL CENTER	13000 BRUCE B DI	TAMPA	FL	33612	HILLSBOROUGH	8139722000	52	64	60	45	75	
10065F	W PALM BEACH VA MEDICAL CENTER	7305 N. MILITARY	WEST PALM BEAC	FL	33410	PALM BEACH	5614228600	49	65	56	43	71	
11030F	AUGUSTA VA MEDICAL CENTER	1 FREEDOM WAY	AUGUSTA	GA	30904	RICHMOND	7068232201	52	62	60	62	78	
11029F	DECATUR (ATLANTA) VA MEDICAL CE	1670 CLAIRMONT	DECATUR	GA	30033	DEKALB	4043216111	53	62	64	60	80	
11031F	DUBLIN VA MEDICAL CENTER	1826 VETERANS B	DUBLIN	GA	31021	LAURENS	4782772701	58	77	71	76	80	
16003F	VA CENTRAL IOWA HEALTHCARE SYS	3600 30TH STREET	DES MOINES	IA	50310	POLK	5156995999	59	75	64	56	77	
16004F	IOWA CITY VA HEALTHCARE SYSTEM	601 HIGHWAY 6 V	IOWA CITY	IA	52246	JOHNSON	3193380581	56	74	68	66	75	
13003F	BOISE VA MEDICAL CENTER	500 W. FORT STRE	BOISE	ID	83702	ADA	2084221000	55	72	68	60	81	

FIGURE 3.2 Levels of measurement.

3.2.2 Descriptive Statistics

As a precursor to analysis of data and conducting tests, getting basic information on the data distribution and being cognizant of the level of measurement is a good starting point. Within Excel, there are a variety of statistical functions that can be invoked to run descriptive statistics on variables of

Tutorial video for Section 3.2.2 is available by accessing the following url: https://connect .springerpub.com/content/book/978-0-8261-5028-8/chapter/ch11

interest. Rather than spending time and effort in running separate measures of central tendency, variation, skewness, and kurtosis, consider using the Analysis ToolPak to more efficiently get descriptive statistics.

In the worksheet with HCAHPS survey data from VA facilities, click on "Data" in the menu bar and in the ribbon, click on "Data Analysis"—at the far right of the ribbon (Figure 3.3). In the "Data Analysis" panel, scroll and choose "Descriptive Statistics." Next, to get descriptive statistics on the variable "understood care," we need to click on the "up arrow" next to "Input Range" and select the entire column of data on "Understood Care," including the first row containing the label. Make sure to select "Column" for "Grouped By" as the data are in a column. The default output option is to provide the descriptive statistics in a new worksheet. Before clicking on "OK" make sure to check the box for "Summary Statistics."

Click on the new worksheet where the descriptive statistics output is. After resizing the first column, you will see that a comprehensive list of descriptive statistics for "Understood Care" has been generated (Figure 3.4). Let us understand the various measures of central tendency included in the descriptive statistics output. Since Excel like any other statistical software is agnostic to measurement level, consider the measurement level of the variable to determine the appropriate descriptive statistics to use. In this case, for the variable "Understood Care," since this is at the interval/ratio level, we can report the mean or the median of the data as its measure of central tendency. The mode or the most commonly occurring value in the data is rarely used as another measure of central tendency. In developing confidence intervals and testing hypotheses about the mean, we will be using the standard error of the mean (see Chapter 4, Setting Bounds for Healthcare Data and Hypothesis Testing Using Excel®). The standard deviation and the variance are measures of dispersion or spread in the data while the skewness and kurtosis also help to describe other aspects of how the data is distributed. These four measures that describe the distribution are useful for determining if the assumptions for undertaking detailed statistical analysis are met or not. The range denotes the difference between the maximum and minimum values of the data and is a simpler measure of dispersion in data. The last two output entries in descriptive statistics are the sum and the count. As the name suggests, "sum" is just summarizing all the values of the variable "Understood Care" and the "count" denotes how many cases there are containing values for this variable.

At a minimum, reporting a central tendency and using the standard error to compute confidence interval around the mean (see Chapter 4, Setting Bounds for Healthcare Data and Hypothesis Testing Using Excel®) is a good practice. Other measures of dispersion as well as description of the distribution are used when we want to run detailed statistical analysis and want to ensure that assumptions about the distribution of data are met.

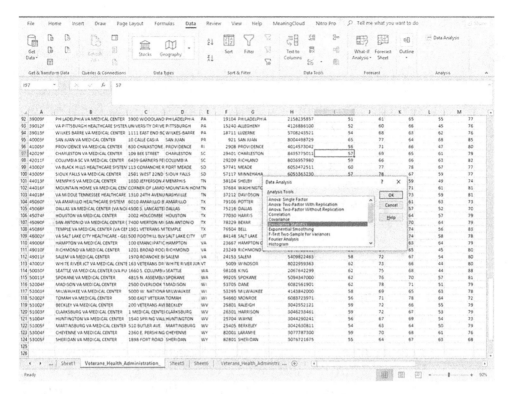

FIGURE 3.3 Descriptive statistics using Analysis ToolPak.

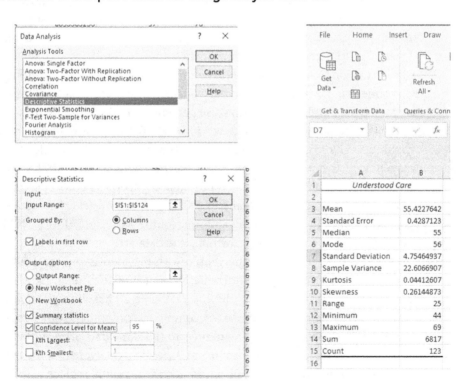

FIGURE 3.4 Descriptive statistics input and output.

3.2.3 Frequency Distribution

The descriptive statistics routine in Excel helps to bring out key measures about our data. Together with these descriptive statistics, we can also summarize vast amounts of data using a frequency distribution. Consider the variable "Understood Care." In using descriptive statistics in Excel (see "Descriptive Statistics" earlier), we report the minimum and maximum values in our data on "Understood Care." Within the bounds of these minimum and maximum values, the frequency or number of times each data value occurs provides useful information about our data.

To get started with using the formula for frequency distribution, we need to make some decisions. We know our minimum and maximum values. However, we need to now decide what criteria we are going to use to form intervals and how many intervals we are going to create between the minimum and maximum values. There are no hard and fast rules for most variables except for age groups and income categories where you could pick the standard intervals for ages. The criteria for creating intervals should be based on the question that you are trying to answer. For instance, since this variable is like the traditional Hospital Consumer Assessment of Healthcare Providers and Systems (HCAHPS) that have star ratings ranging from one to five stars, we could attempt to create star ratings here. The traditional HCAHPS star ratings are determined based on complex criteria and computations that take into consideration the scores on periodically completed surveys by patients and based on which cutoffs are determined for each of the composite variables to determine star ratings. Since the HCAHPS from the Veterans Administration (VA) are not included in this computation, we can attempt to determine star ratings for VA HCAHPS. A good starting point for this is to determine percentiles and possibly use percentiles to determine star ratings.

Having decided on how to create intervals between our minimum and maximum values, we need to identify each of the cutoff percentiles for our frequency distribution. In Figure 3.5, we have typed each of the cutoffs (10th, 20th, …, 100th). In the column adjacent to these cutoff percentiles, we need to determine the actual cutoff data points for each of these identified percentiles. To do so, we use the percentile formula "=PERCENTILE. EXC($E$2:$E$124,0.1)." In this formula, the data array is in cells E2 to E124 and the comma separates the percentile with 0.1 identifying the 10th percentile. A modification in this formula is the use of the dollar signs in the data array. This serves to make the cell reference an absolute cell reference such that when we copy this down the column to compute the other remaining percentiles, the formula will still refer to the same data array and we just need to change the percentile from 0.1 to 0.2 and so on. Note that for the last percentile—100th, rather than using the formula, simply replace it with the maximum value. These percentile cutoffs that we just computed create bins for which the frequency distribution is computed in Excel. For instance, the first cutoff of 49 creates a bin (or interval) from the minimum value of 44 to the cutoff of 49. The next bin has a cutoff of 51.8 and creates a bin (or interval) from greater than 49 to 51.8 and so on. "Bins" are the nomenclature used by Excel for the formula for computing frequencies.

Once the bin values have been identified or created, we are ready to do the computation of frequencies. To do this, we need the frequencies to appear in the adjacent cells in the next column (see Figure 3.5). Go ahead and select these cells, making sure to select one additional cell in this adjacent cell. Since we have 10 bins, we select all 10 adjacent cells in the next column and select one more cell down. With these cells highlighted, go ahead and enter the formula for computing frequencies "=FREQUENCY(E2:E124,I2:I11)." This formula has two parts, the first part identifies the data array or location of the data (E2:E124) and the second part separated by a comma identifies the bins that we created (I2:I11). The computation of frequencies is an array formula in Excel, that is, the computation of this formula appears in more than one cell. In order to have the computations of frequencies appear in the cells corresponding to the bins, we need to simultaneously hold down "CTRL" and "Shift" keys and press "Enter." If you merely press "Enter" the frequency will be computed only in one cell. Since we correctly applied the frequency formula as an array formula (simultaneously held down "CTRL" and "Shift" keys before pressing

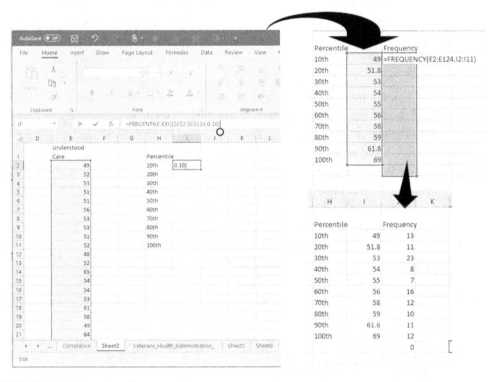

FIGURE 3.5 Running frequencies.

"Enter") we get the frequency computed for each of the bins. The extra cell that we included for this computation, which does not have a corresponding bin, is to ensure that we have covered all data points—hence the "0."

Once computed, the frequencies with their bins are available. Depending on how we decide to have star ratings, these bins and percentiles can be used to figure out how many VA facilities have what specific star ratings. Just like this, for any other data, based on the specific question that is to be answered, we can define and create bins and compute frequencies using this array formula in Excel.

3.3 Using Pivot Tables

Variables at the interval and ratio level of measurement are well suited to summarizing data using tables. For this level of measurement, pivot tables are a powerful and adaptive functionality that quickly helps to analyze raw data and discern underlying patterns and trends. This feature of Excel appears complicated the first time you see it in operation. Its versatility is worth the pain in familiarizing yourself with how pivot tables work and using them. A word of caution in using pivot tables: Pivot tables are not easily used by all forms of data. They are best suited to data that can be summarized in rows and columns—for example, health expenditure data, number of visits, number of procedures, number of health providers or facilities, and so on. However, for data such as mortality rates, health outcomes, coverage rates, and so on, additional mastery of advanced features in pivot tables will certainly help.

To explore basic features of pivot tables, we will use historical data on national health expenditure by source of funds in the United States. These data are available through the CMS as an Excel file and span the years 1960 through 2016 (CMS, 2018). To focus on the functionality of pivot tables, the subcategories of the different sources of funds have been removed from this file. Open Dataset 8. Click on any cell containing data and then select "Insert" from the toolbar and choose the first option here "Pivot Table" (see Figure 3.6). You will notice that the second option here is "Recommended Pivot Tables." Under the second option, based on the nature of data, Excel narrows the choices for creating pivot tables. We will use the "Pivot Tables" options to gain familiarity with the basic features of pivot tables. Go ahead and select "Pivot Tables," whence, a dialog box opens. Within this dialog box there are two options that need our attention. The first, "Choose the data that you want to analyze" should already be chosen—as evidenced by the selection of table/range bounded by dashed lines. Only if the data are not selected, make sure to click the "up arrow" next to "table/range" and select the entire range of data. For the second option—"Choose where you want the Pivot Table report to be placed"—choose "New Worksheet." A new

---

worksheet is now revealed (Figure 3.7) with two distinct parts—a blank worksheet with directions to create a report by choosing from the pivot table field list and a vertical section labeled "pivot table fields." A closer examination of the pivot table fields shows that the columns from our original data on national health expenditure are displayed here as fields. Below these fields are four quadrants—filters, columns, values, and rows. We will be placing the fields from our pivot table fields in these quadrants to summarize the data. Depending on the choice of fields and the quadrants used, our summary report of the pivot table will vary. The most elementary pivot table report can be created by choosing one field either as a row or column and choosing the other field as a value.

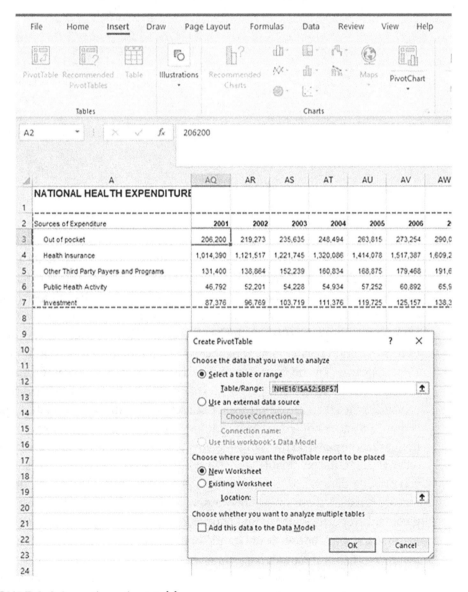

FIGURE 3.6 Inserting pivot tables.

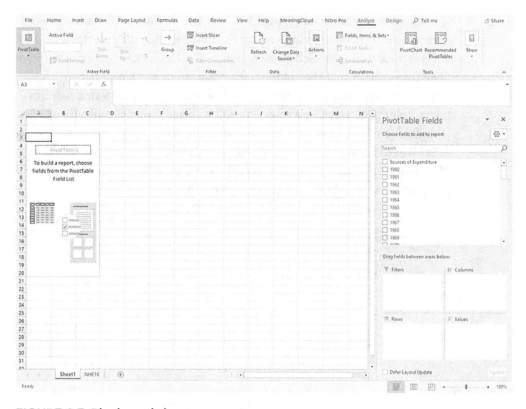

FIGURE 3.7 Blank worksheet.

To create our first pivot table summary report, go ahead and hover your mouse over "Source of Expenditure" from the section "Pivot Table Fields" and left-click and drag this field to the "Rows" quadrant. Immediately you will see the Summary Table Report rows populated with the unique sources of expenditure. Next, using your mouse as just described—hover and right click—drag the year "1960" from "Pivot Table Fields" to the "Values" quadrant. This action results in national health expenditure figures in millions for 1960 appearing in the Summary Table Report. Now go ahead and use the same procedure to bring the years 1961 and 1962 to the "Values" quadrant.

So far, other than providing a small subset of the data, the pivot table report (Figure 3.8) does not appear to be adding any additional value. Also, you will notice that the panel on the right—"Pivot Table Fields"—has disappeared. Click on any data in the pivot table report and the panel on the right appears. While you are in a data cell in this report, go ahead and right-click. In the options that are revealed, there are several ways to modify the values represented in the pivot table report. Go ahead and choose "Show Values As" and from the submenu that opens choose "% of Grand Total." These steps have altered the summary report (not the underlying data) to show percentage of national health expenditure (Grand Total) for the different sources of funds. Go ahead and repeat these steps to display the other 2 years in percentage terms.

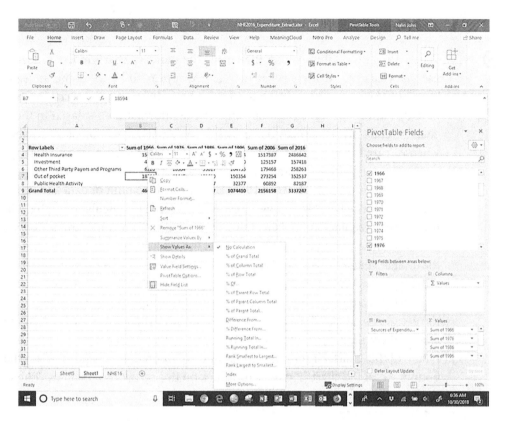

FIGURE 3.8 Pivot tables.

In case there are other categories for sources of funds included in the raw underlying data, such as regions, these would appear in the pivot table fields and can be used either as columns or placed under the "Sources of Expenditure" as subcategories. Alternately, if these subcategories are placed in rows above "Sources of Expenditure," this will lead to the categories being the first rows and "Sources of Expenditure" as the subcategory. The order in which fields are placed in rows determines which is the row and which is the subcategory.

Getting back to the pivot table report,u choose any data cell and right-click to reveal options. One of the displayed options is "Show Details." Since this report is a summary report, "Show Details" takes you to the underlying data for the specific cell chosen in this summary report. If for instance, data on "Investments" for 1962 is chosen and we choose "Details," the underlying data on Investments for all years are brought up in a separate sheet.

Pivot tables make it easy to choose specific fields (columns of data) to be included in the Summary Table Report. Thus, even though we have 50 years of data, we can choose specific years in the fields to display. For instance, if we want data for every decade from 1966, it is as simple as providing tick marks for the specific decades in the fields list. Since the year fields contain values, they will populate the "Values" quadrant and are displayed as columns in our Summary Table Report.

3.4 Pivot Charts

When using pivot tables, rather than using the standard charts in Excel, always use pivot charts. Pivot charts at first glance appear to be the same as regular charts. However, in addition to having the features of regular charts, they have dynamic capabilities to easily change the information displayed in these charts. Access pivot charts by using "Insert" or "Analyze" section of the toolbar when you are in a sheet containing the Summary Table Report for a pivot table.

Continuing with the example already presented, we have just included year values at 10-year intervals from 1966. Go into each column of data and right-click any data cell and in "Show Value As" choose "No Calculation." This will revert the percentages to dollar values. Once all data values are now as dollars, go ahead and invoke pivot charts through the "Insert" or "Analyze" section of the toolbar (Figure 3.9). For displaying the data, you can now choose any of the chart types and options that are available. Let us go ahead and choose for now the clustered columns. The choice of clustered columns shows the pattern over the decades within each source of national health expenditure. Notice that the clustered columns look like a standard chart in Excel. To access the dynamic nature of this chart, click on the arrow next to "Source of Expenditure" on the bottom left of the chart (Figure 3.10). Click on this arrow and uncheck "Public

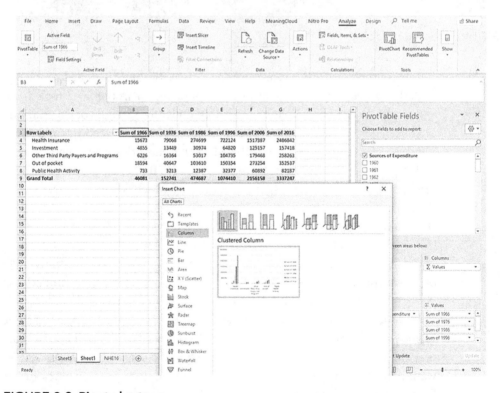

FIGURE 3.9 Pivot charts.

Tutorial video for Section 3.4 is available by accessing the following url: https://connect .springerpub.com/content/book/978-0-8261-5028-8/chapter/ch11

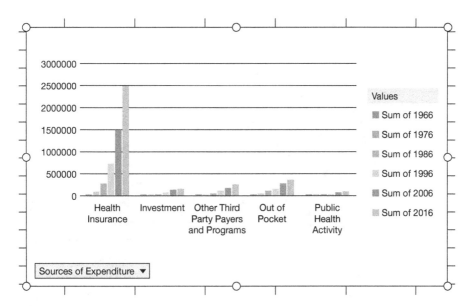

FIGURE 3.10 Dynamic pivot charts.

Health Activity." Immediately, the columns related to "Public Health Activity" are removed from both the pivot chart as well as the pivot table.

Right-clicking on your pivot chart brings up options to alter your chart as well as format options. One of the options here is to "Select Data." This option is also available through regular charts in Excel and choosing this option, options up another menu prompting you to switch rows and columns (Figure 3.11). Use this menu to switch rows and columns. Right-click once more on the pivot chart and bring up the option to "Change Chart Type." Here choose a Line Chart. In the resulting chart, the focus is now clearly on visualizing the pattern over the years in each of these sources of national health expenditure, and the rapid increase in health insurance as a key source of funding for national health expenditure is evident. Moving from the clustered columns changes the focus in visualization from intra (within sources of expenditure) to inter (across sources of expenditure).

Another feature within pivot tables in Excel is the ability to group rows of data. For the current example, we just switched rows and columns and thus have sums of years in the rows. We will go ahead and right-click within the pivot chart and "Select Data" and again switch rows and columns such that we are back where we started with Sources of Expenditure in rows. Go ahead and place your cursor in the pivot table and choose "Analyze" from the toolbar. Toward the middle is an option to "Group" (Figure 3.12). We notice in our data that two sources of expenditure, public health activity and investments, are relatively small compared to the other categories. We can group these two categories by clicking on one source of expenditure (public health activity) and then holding down the control key and using the mouse to click on the next row (investment). Since the two sources of expenditure were not in adjacent rows, we used the control key to select non-contiguous cells. If the cells were in contiguous rows, we could have

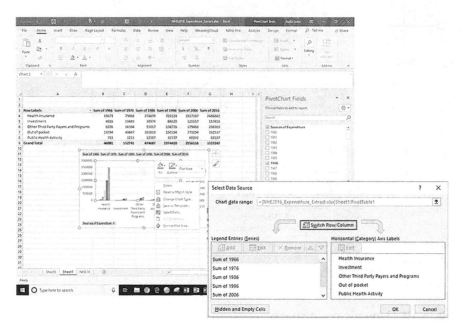

FIGURE 3.11 Switching rows and columns in chart.

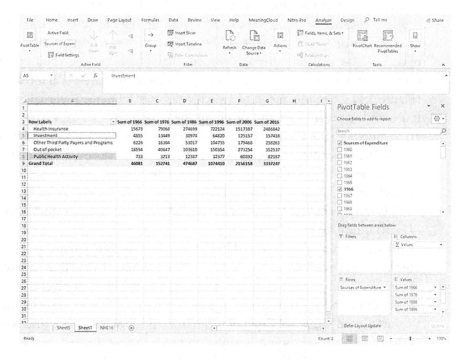

FIGURE 3.12 Grouping rows in pivot tables and charts.

also held down the shift key and selected all contiguous rows. Anyway, once the rows are selected, go back to the "Group" option under "Analyze" in the toolbar and choose "Group Selection." Now Public Health and Investment are shown both as a group as well as separately within the group. You will also notice that the remaining categories in this pivot table have also now been created as groups of one. You can go ahead and group any of the remaining sources of expenditure as other groups. Click on "Group1" (grouping of Public Health Activity and Investment) and you can overwrite this group name to something more relatable, such as "Investment and Public Health." In the pivot table and pivot chart (in case one is open), you notice that there are two sources of expenditure—one ungrouped and the other grouped. To clear your display as well as declutter the table, go into the pivot table (chart) fields. In this panel, under the "Rows" quadrant you will notice two rows of Sources of Expenditure. The ungrouped original sources of expenditure are in the bottom row and the grouped sources of expenditure are in the top row. To remove the ungrouped sources of expenditure, simply choose the bottom row in the pivot table (chart) field and drag it and drop it on the worksheet. Now the pivot table and chart have a cleaner feel to them. "Groups" are a great tool to collapse categories that are outliers and may distract attention away from patterns in data on which you want to focus.

3.5 Using Chart Types in Excel

Thus far we have covered pivot charts that are unique to use of pivot tables. Remember that pivot charts are similar in many respects to regular charts—except for the dynamic features that allow you to choose and remove specific categories from both the pivot charts as well as pivot tables. In this section, we will cover the use of most (common and uncommon) chart types in newer versions of Excel (2016 and beyond).

Since this is a discussion of charts in general that can also be applied to pivot tables and charts, we will continue to work with the pivot tables that were just created in Excel in the previous section. These chart features can also be accessed when you are in any worksheet in Excel. To access charts, first highlight the data that you want to display in your chart, click on "Insert" in the toolbar and then choose the "down arrow" near "Chart" (Figure 3.13). In the menu that opens there are two tabs—"Recommended Charts" and "All Charts." Based on the type of data in the worksheet, Excel narrows down to the chart suitable to your data. Since we are exploring the use of charts, go ahead and click on "All Charts." In each chart, you can undertake a variety of customizations as well as invoke several features such as editing and formatting the chart elements (title, legends, axes, labels, etc.). One especially useful feature is to ensure that you include data labels in the chart. Data labels include the actual value on the chart and you and the reader do not have to second guess yourself as to the value. Invoke this feature by hovering over the chart with your mouse till you see a "data series" label with value pop up. Right click in the chart and choose "Add data label" to display the value on the chart. Be judicious in your use of data labels and ensure that you have not included so many data labels that they overlap on the chart. We will use this procedure

Tutorial video for Sections 3.5 to 3.5.2 is available by accessing the following url: https://connect.springerpub.com/content/book/978-0-8261-5028-8/chapter/ch11

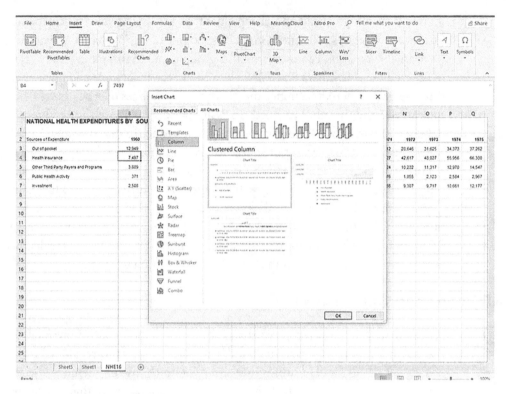

FIGURE 3.13 Accessing charts in Excel.

to access "All Charts" and then go to specific chart types in the following subsections that describe data types and situations when particular chart types are suitable. A table of each chart type and considerations in their use is included in the summary section at the end of this chapter.

3.5.1 Column Charts

Column charts are a useful chart type to show changes in categories over time. In this example, it shows how the different sources of expenditure have changed over six decades selected. In order to use column charts, your data table should have row categories (sources of expenditure) and several columns of data (expenditure over the years). Highlight the entire table and access charts through "Insert" on the toolbar and then choose the "down arrow" next to "Charts." In the menu that opens, choose the tab for "All Charts" and "Column." In this clustered column chart (Figure 3.14A) the sources of expenditure are on the x-axis and the values on the y-axis with the display showing how each source of expenditure has changed over time. The rapid increase in health insurance as a major source of national health expenditure is highlighted in this chart type.

3.5.2 Line Charts

Line charts are useful to compare categories over time. Unlike column charts which focus on changes over time within the same category, line charts compare categories across time. We will use the same example as before as a line chart. Navigate to "All Charts" using the general procedure described earlier (Using Charts in Excel), and choose line charts. In the display, you will notice that the categories are on the x-axis and the values are on the y-axis and the display does not seem right—the lines should be the categories and not the values. We need to switch the data rows and columns in order to display the categories on the y-axis and the values on the x-axis. Right click on the chart and choose "Select Data" (Figure 3.14B). In the menu that opens, click on "Switch Rows/

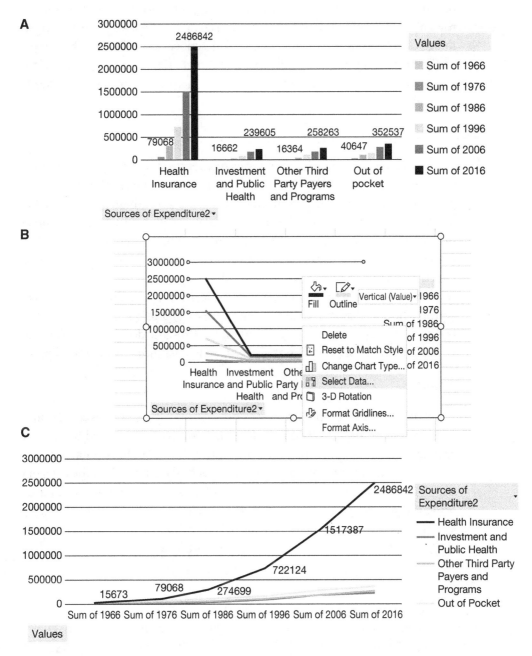

FIGURE 3.14 Column and line charts in Excel.

Columns" and the display changes. Now the categories are on the y-axis and the data values are on the x-axis and the chart compares the trend over time in each of the sources of national health expenditure (Figure 3.14C).

3.5.3 Pie Charts

(▶) If the relationship of part to whole is the question, pie charts are a great way to represent this relationship. This especially works well if we have categories and only one series of data. In our example, it would be the different sources of national health expenditure and values for one point in time. Go ahead and choose the rows of "Source of Expenditure" and select a column of data (say 1966). Navigate to "All Charts" using the general procedure described earlier (Using Chart Types in Excel), and choose pie charts. In the pie chart (Figure 3.15A), each of the sources of national health expenditure is shown as a proportion of national health expenditure.

3.5.4 Doughnut

For the pie chart, displaying one series of data for a few categories (sources of expenditure) works well. In case you want to show the relationship of proportion to whole for two or more data series (more than 1 year of data), consider a doughnut. For this example, we will choose the rows of sources of expenditure and all data series (1966 through 2016). Navigate to "All Charts" using the general procedure described earlier (Using Chart Types in Excel), and choose pie and, within that, the doughnut. In the doughnut chart (Figure 3.15B), each of the sources of national health expenditure is shown as a proportion of national health expenditure as a band and each year of data is shown as a separate band of the doughnut. Thus, the doughnut chart facilitates comparison of proportions of sources of expenditure over several years.

3.5.5 Bar Chart

(▶) A bar chart is like a column chart and provides the same visualization—comparison of how individual categories (sources of expenditure) have changed over time. The difference is that bar charts are horizontal, and the column charts are vertical. Bar charts are especially useful when the category names are very long. Select the entire table of data and navigate to "All Charts" using the general procedure described earlier (Using Chart Types in Excel), and choose bar charts. In the bar chart (Figure 3.16A), changes over time in each of the sources of national health expenditure are the focus.

(▶) Tutorial video for Sections 3.5.3 to 3.5.4 is available by accessing the following url: https://connect.springerpub.com/content/book/978-0-8261-5028-8/chapter/ch11

(▶) Tutorial video for Sections 3.5.5 to 3.5.6 is available by accessing the following url: https://connect.springerpub.com/content/book/978-0-8261-5028-8/chapter/ch11

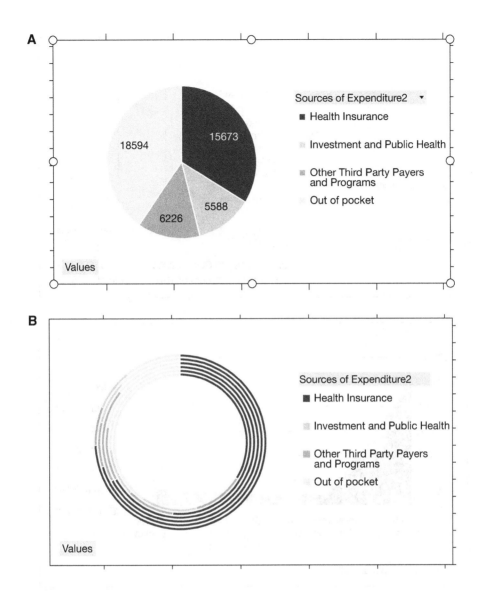

FIGURE 3.15 Pie charts and doughnut charts.

3.5.6 Area Chart

An area chart is like a line chart and provides the same visualization—comparison of how categories (sources of expenditure) have changed over time and adds a comparison of proportion through use of area under the line. Go ahead and choose the entire table and navigate to charts and choose area chart. In the display (Figure 3.16B), you will notice that the categories are on the x-axis and the values are on the y-axis and the display does not seem right—the lines should be the categories and not the values. We need to switch the data rows and columns in order to display the categories on the y-axis and the values on the x-axis. Right click on the chart and choose "Select Data." In the menu that opens, click on "Switch Rows/Columns" and the display changes. Now the

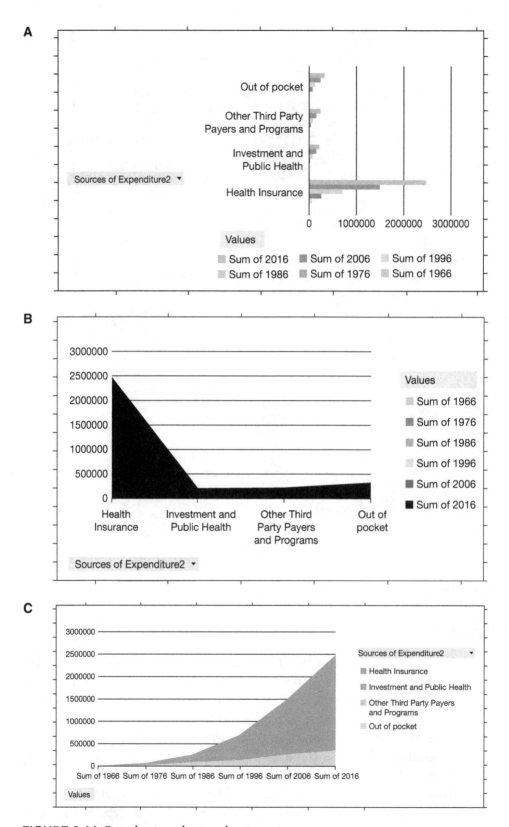

FIGURE 3.16 Bar chart and area chart.

categories are on the y-axis and the data values are on the x-axis and the chart compares the trend over time in each of the sources of national health expenditure (Figure 3.16C). By filling the area under each line, it also visually provides cues to the proportions of each source of expenditure to national expenditure.

3.5.7 Radar

A radar looks like a spider web and shows if data in three to seven categories (sources of expenditure) are equal contributors to the total (national health expenditure). This radar chart is more suited to data that is not constrained by pivot tables, so we will go into the overall historical data on national health expenditure. Select the rows of sources of expenditure and 5 years of data. Navigate to "All Charts" using the general procedure described earlier (Using Chart Types in Excel), and choose "radar." The radar chart shows with two options. The first one has the years as the vertices and the sources of expenditure as the series while the second has the sources of expenditure as the vertices and the years as the series. Choose the second option (Figure 3.17A). With the sources of expenditures as vertices, you can see on a year-to-year basis how unequal the individual sources of expenditure are with out-of-pocket expenses far exceeding other sources of expenditure in the early 1960s.

3.5.8 Tree Map

A tree map is like a pie chart and provides a comparison of each component category (sources of expenditure) to the whole (national health expenditure). The tree map is not available for pivot tables, so we will go to the overall historical data sheet for national health expenditure. Go ahead and select the sources of expenditure and the first column of data for 1966. Navigate to "All Charts" using the general procedure described earlier (Using Chart Types in Excel), and choose "tree map." The resulting tree map (Figure 3.17B) forces all the sources of expenditure into the square tree map with the areas proportional to the size of each source of expenditure.

3.5.9 Funnel Chart

Funnel charts work well with data that is sorted from highest to lowest value for categories (sources of expenditure) for one column of values. In our example, we have the sources of expenditure and data for 1960. Select this data and sort using "Data" on the toolbar (Figure 3.18). Click on "Sort" and when the Sort Menu

---

Tutorial video for Sections 3.5.7 to 3.5.8 is available by accessing the following url: https://connect.springerpub.com/content/book/978-0-8261-5028-8/chapter/ch11

Tutorial video for Section 3.5.9 is available by accessing the following url: https://connect.springerpub.com/content/book/978-0-8261-5028-8/chapter/ch11

A

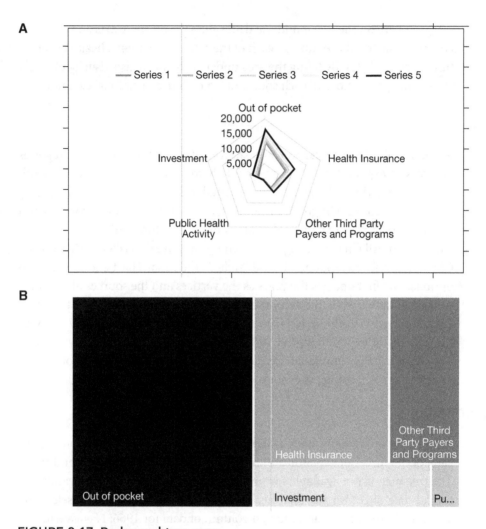

FIGURE 3.17 Radar and tree map.

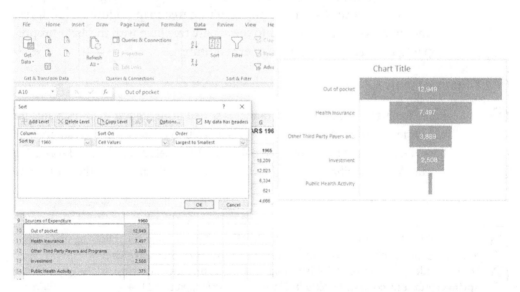

FIGURE 3.18 Sorting data and creating funnel charts.

opens up, make sure to check "My data has headers" and choose 1960 for "Sort by" and "Order" as "Largest to Smallest." Once the data are sorted, select this data. Navigate to "All Charts" using the general procedure described earlier (Using Chart Types in Excel), and choose "funnel." In the funnel chart, the sources of expenditure are stacked as in a funnel from highest to lowest and the sizes provide a good comparison of contributions of each of these sources of expenditures.

3.5.10 Combo Chart

A combo chart, as the name suggests, provides the flexibility to use two different charts together in the same figure. This is especially useful if you would like to show for categories (source of expenditure) not just the trend over time of annual expenditure amounts but also another value (like an average) for these categories. To show how to create a combo chart, let us continue with our example with the historical national health expenditure values. In our example, we have the annual expenditure amounts for the sources of expenditure for 1996, 2006, and 2016. The last column of data includes the average (1960–2016) for these sources. In order to work with combo charts, we need to ensure that the data table is appropriate with the categories as columns and the values in rows. We can transpose the rows and columns by copying this table and, before pasting in another location on the worksheet, making sure to use the "Paste Options" and use "Transpose." Now that the sources of expenditure are in

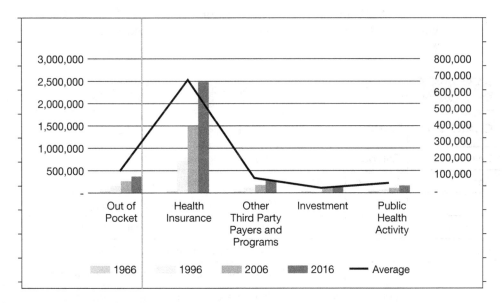

FIGURE 3.19 Combo charts.

Tutorial video for Section 3.5.10 is available by accessing the following url: https://connect .springerpub.com/content/book/978-0-8261-5028-8/chapter/ch11

columns and the values are in rows, go ahead and select this table. Navigate to "All Charts" using the general procedure described earlier (Using Chart Types in Excel), and choose "Combo Chart." In the menu that opens, toward the bottom you will see a panel that has each row of values and an option to choose the chart type for each row of values (Figure 3.19). Make sure to have each of the 3 years as "clustered columns" and average as "line." Since the average values are better represented using a different scale than the one for the yearly values, go ahead and make sure to check the box for "Secondary Axis" for average values. The resulting chart (Figure 3.19) has the values for each of the 3 years as clustered columns and the average values as a line. Since we chose a secondary axis for the average values, the axis for the average values is on the right of the chart. Through this combo chart, we can combine both the pattern over time in the sources of expenditure as well as plot the average values on the same chart.

3.6 Considerations in Using Different Chart Types

Always start with the question that you want to answer and let that guide your choice of chart type. Chart types help you to summarize a tremendous amount of data. In crunching this data, your question that is to be answered must come out clearly. Let that be the driving force and not the artistic quotient of a chart type. In choosing chart types, put yourself in the shoes of your audience and choose simplicity over complexity.

In Table 3.1 there is a quick summary of the key aspects of the chart types in this chapter. This includes what appears on the x- and y-axes (if applicable) as well as key considerations in using a chart type. Take for example the column and line charts. Both contain very similar information and it almost

TABLE 3.1   Considerations in Using Chart Types

CHART TYPE	X-AXIS	Y-AXIS	CONSIDERATION
Column	Category	Value	Two or more data series
Line	Category	Value	Two or more data series
Pie			One data series; part to whole comparison
Doughnut			One or more data series; part to whole comparison
Bar		Category	Comparison among individual items
Area	Category	Value	Show change over time; total value over time
Radar	Value	Value	Compare aggregate value of several data series
Treemap			Compare different categories
Funnel			Show values across multiple stages in process
Combo			Use two or more chart types with different axes

appears that these chart types can be used interchangeably. However, there are subtle differences in these chart types. The column chart focuses attention on each variable and how it is changing over time, while the line chart does a better job at comparing time trends across different variables (see Figure 3.14). Other chart types have more unique applications and Table 3.1, together with the examples of each chart (covered earlier in this chapter) can guide you in making informed choices.

Use Table 3.1 in conjunction with your level of measurement to determine appropriate use of different chart types and remember that there are no hard and fast rules—only pointers on what chart type may work better in particular situations.

3.7 Competency Development

It starts with a question. Yes, that is the secret behind working with data and making sense of what the data is trying to tell us. As identified in Box 3.1, it is very easy to get stuck behind mountains of data. However, having a clear purpose and a message to convey—trends in mortality across time and geography as well as the leading causes of mortality—it is easy to sift through almost 2,000 lines of data and depict the key message through thoughtful graphs and charts. This is what the domain of critical thinking is all about. Especially since we have mountains of data to sift through as well as several sources of healthcare data, it is important to spend time thinking through the question that needs to be answered before diving into the data.

Having identified question(s) that are sought to be answered and obtaining data, we are ready to systematically proceed through this process by coming to terms with the levels of measurement—nominal, ordinal, interval, and ratio—that our data variables are in. For variables at nominal or ordinal levels of measurement, frequency and percent distributions are appropriate, while interval and ratio levels of measurements are well suited to a variety of tables, charts, and statistics (Singleton & Straits, 2010). Proceeding thus, we use skills and applications from the competency domains of information management and critical thinking. Then, the use of descriptive statistics and frequency distributions to provide elementary information about data distributions begins our foray into the competency domain of communication.

Next, gaining familiarity with the pivot tables routine in Excel is a good way to summarize information from variables at the interval and ratio level. Pivot tables are then a stepping stone to pivot charts which add dynamic capabilities to regular charts in Excel. Using both the pivot tables and pivot charts in conjunction adds versatility to the process of summarizing and depicting information. In summarizing and focusing on key parts of the data through tables and charts, it is then possible to monitor progress on these variables. These routines further extend the application of skills from the competency domains of information management, performance management, as well as communication.

Our ability to summarize information through charts is enhanced through exposure to nine specific chart types and one combination chart type in Excel. Each of these chart types has applications in specific situations such as to emphasize patterns, trends, or comparison. Understanding when to use these chart types further reinforces the competency domains of performance management and communication.

In this chapter, by ensuring that the starting point for summarizing and presenting data is the questions behind healthcare decision-making, we ensure that application of skills in the critical thinking domain are addressed. Next, by relying on the levels of measurement of data to inform both the summary and presentation of data, the focus is on skill development in critical thinking, information management, and communication. Finally, by becoming conversant with the different chart types in Excel and considerations as to when to use specific chart types, application and skill development in performance management and communication domains are emphasized.

3.8 Summary

The starting point for summarizing and presenting data is developing and clarifying questions that the data can help answer. These questions are based on decisions that we need to make in healthcare. Given the volumes of data that are now available, ways to summarize this data, including presenting this data through graphs and charts, are also informed by the levels of measurement in data. Within Excel, healthcare data are presented through a variety of graphs and charts. However, these graphs and charts are not an end in themselves and should help to answer the questions behind healthcare decision-making.

3.9 Discussion Questions

3.9.1   What are the issues that you consider in deciding how to present your data?

3.9.2   Think of examples from healthcare of data at nominal or ordinal level of measurement. How would you summarize or present these data?

3.9.3   Think of examples from healthcare of data at interval or ratio level of measurement. How would you summarize or present these data?

3.9.4   When looking for ways to display your data, toward which do you lean—tables or graphs? Why?

3.9.5   What issues would you consider in choosing between a bar graph and a pie chart?

3.10 Practice Problems

All datasets required for the practice problems are available for download at http://connect.springerpub.com/content/book/978-0-8261-5028-8.

3.10.1 Dataset 6 contains data on national health expenditures for the period 2001–2016. You have been tasked by a senator's office to summarize data for 2001 and 2016. Develop a plan for how you would go about summarizing this data and provide a summary for 2001 and 2016.

3.10.2 The senator's office comes back to you with another request. With an upcoming committee hearing on health, the senator would like you to provide a summary of Medicare and Private Health Insurance expenditure for the period 2001–2016. Use Dataset 6 to develop a plan for how you would go about summarizing this data and provide a summary for Medicare and Private Health Insurance.

3.10.3 For an upcoming debate on national health expenditure, the senator's office would like you to develop a visually appealing display of national health expenditure, private health insurance, and Medicare. Use Dataset 6 to develop a visually appealing and informative display for the senator's office.

3.10.4 The senator's office promises that this is the last request. In order to be better prepared for discussing national health expenditure, the senator's office would like you to draw a comparison of health insurance and the proportion spent on Medicare and private health insurance. Use Dataset 6 to develop this comparison.

3.10.5 Continuing your role as the analyst with the health advocacy group. Dataset 5 contains data that need to be presented to your team. You have been tasked by your Team Lead to look at two fields—column F (Premature Death Value) and column K (Poor or Fair Health Value).

a. What considerations will you be mindful of as you start to look at this data and prepare it for presentation?

b. Use a pivot table to summarize information on these two fields at the state level.

c. Prepare a chart that shows a comparison of five states with the highest premature death value.

d. Prepare another chart that shows average poor or fair health value.

e. Summarize the key points from your data analysis and display.

Tutorial videos provided for Practice Problems 3.10.1—3.10.7 can be accessed by accessing the following url: https://connect.springerpub.com/content/book/978-0-8261-5028-8/chapter/ch11

3.10.6 The VA has just received Dataset 3 that contains the HCAHPS scores for VA facilities. You have been tasked by your Team Lead to look at three fields—column J (rating 9 or 10), column L (Room Quiet at Night) and column S (Recommend Hospital).

a. What considerations will you be mindful of as you start to look at this data and prepare it for presentation?

b. Prepare a chart that shows a comparison of these three variables across states.

c. Summarize what this comparison of variables reveals.

3.10.7 With the continuing changes in healthcare reform, there is renewed interest in looking at the early effects of the Affordable Care Act. Dataset 9 contains information on changes in the uninsured rate from 2010 to 2015 in each state. What specific question can you ask using this data and how would you present this data to answer your question?

See Chapter 11, Video Tutorials and Answers to Practice Problems Using Healthcare Datasets in Excel®, for video answers to the practice problems.

References

Centers for Medicare and Medicaid Services. (2016, October 19). Veterans Health Administration hospital performance plan. Retrieved from https://www.cms.gov/Medicare/Quality-Initiatives-Patient-Assessment-Instruments/HospitalQualityInits/VA-Data.html

Centers for Medicare and Medicaid Services. (2018, January 8). National Health Expenditure data: Historical. Retrieved from https://www.cms.gov/Research-Statistics-Data-and-Systems/Statistics-Trends-and-Reports/NationalHealthExpendData/NationalHealthAccountsHistorical.html

Keller, D. K. (2006). *The tao of statistics: A path to understanding (with no math)*. Thousand Oaks, CA: Sage Publications.

Schutt, R. K. (2015). *Investigating the social world: The process and practice of research* (8th ed.). Thousand Oaks, CA: Sage Publications.

Singleton, R., & Straits, B. C. (2010). *Approaches to social research* (5th ed.). New York, NY: Oxford University Press.

Tableau. (n.d.). Visual analysis best practices: A guidebook. Retrieved from https://www.tableau.com/learn/whitepapers/tableau-visual-guidebook

Tejada-Vera, B. (2019). Leading causes of death: United States, 1999–2017. National Center for Health Statistics. Retrieved from https://www.cdc.gov/nchs/data-visualization/mortality-leading-causes/index_2.htm

4

SETTING BOUNDS FOR HEALTHCARE DATA AND HYPOTHESIS TESTING USING EXCEL®

LEARNING OBJECTIVES

- Acknowledge uncertainty in sampled data
- Compute bounds around estimates to develop confidence intervals
- Differentiate between sample estimates and population values
- Use hypothesis testing to test sample mean using confidence intervals
- Use hypothesis testing to test sample mean using Z-test
- Use hypothesis testing to compare two samples using Z-test

In this chapter, we use Excel to establish 95% confidence intervals around measures of sample data and then use these bounds for testing hypothesis about the underlying population. These steps lead to undertaking Z-test for testing hypotheses about the population mean and comparing two samples. In this chapter, the competency domains of critical thinking, problem-solving, and performance management are emphasized.

4.1 Introduction

In the County Health Rankings (see Box 4.1) we have a ready application of setting bounds on measures as well as setting the stage for computing Z-scores. Using confidence interval, we acknowledge the lack of certainty in point estimates from sample data and use bounds to have greater certainty

---

Throughout the chapter supplemental content is available for the datasets and tutorial videos. Video availability is denoted with an icon. To gain access to these items, please visit the following urls:

Datasets: https://connect.springerpub.com/content/book/978-0-8261-5028-8

⊙ Tutorial Videos: https://connect.springerpub.com/content/book/978-0-8261-5028-8/chapter/ch11

BOX 4.1 COUNTY HEALTH RANKING: CONFIDENCE INTERVALS AND Z-SCORES

The Robert Wood Johnson (RWJ) Foundation has a long-standing commitment to helping understand social and demographic data and determinants of population health. Since 2011 they have partnered with the University of Wisconsin's Population Health Institute to provide the County Health Rankings (County Health Rankings and Roadmaps, n.d.) that aggregates data from a variety of sources and makes available for practitioners, policy makers, and researchers these data and a variety of analytical tools and visualizations as well as the possibility of downloading these data for use.

Within the County Health Rankings, the data are provided as raw data as well as their 95% confidence intervals and Z-scores, where available. In Figure 4.1, a snapshot of the 2018 County Health Rankings for New Jersey is provided. Notice that the county and state level Years of Potential Life Lost Rate includes the lower and upper level 95% confidence interval bounds as well as the Z-scores. In order to better understand these measures, let us consider the measures reported for Atlantic County in New Jersey (Figure 4.1). The Years of Potential Life Lost

FIPS	State	County	Years of Potential Life Lost Rate	95% CI - Low	95% CI - High	Z-Score
34000	New Jersey		5469	5415	5524	
34001	New Jersey	Atlantic	7454	7083	7825	0.99
34003	New Jersey	Bergen	3859	3716	4003	-1.35
34005	New Jersey	Burlington	5797	5540	6054	-0.09
34007	New Jersey	Camden	7464	7195	7734	1.00
34009	New Jersey	Cape May	8288	7556	9020	1.53
34011	New Jersey	Cumberland	8322	7826	8817	1.55
34013	New Jersey	Essex	7103	6894	7311	0.76
34015	New Jersey	Gloucester	6537	6206	6869	0.39
34017	New Jersey	Hudson	4953	4775	5131	-0.64
34019	New Jersey	Hunterdon	4219	3777	4662	-1.11
34021	New Jersey	Mercer	6064	5776	6352	0.09
34023	New Jersey	Middlesex	4311	4158	4465	-1.05
34025	New Jersey	Monmouth	5088	4881	5295	-0.55
34027	New Jersey	Morris	3911	3712	4110	-1.31
34029	New Jersey	Ocean	6398	6163	6632	0.30
34031	New Jersey	Passaic	5545	5321	5769	-0.25
34033	New Jersey	Salem	8843	7981	9704	1.89
34035	New Jersey	Somerset	3904	3657	4150	-1.32
34037	New Jersey	Sussex	5460	5006	5915	-0.31
34039	New Jersey	Union	5035	4826	5244	-0.58
34041	New Jersey	Warren	6020	5446	6594	0.06

FIGURE 4.1 Snapshot of 2018 County Health Ranking: New Jersey.
SOURCE: Retrieved from https://www.countyhealthrankings.org/explore-health-rankings/rankings-data-documentation

(continued)

BOX 4.1 (*continued*)

Rate in Atlantic County, New Jersey is 7,454 per 100,000. These data are collected and reported by the National Center for Health Statistics, Centers for Disease Control and Prevention (CDC). Since this measure is reported based on mortality files submitted by health entities, there is a certain lack of certainty about this exact figure. In order to account for this uncertainty, the standard deviation and the related standard error of the mean are used (see "Setting Bounds on Data" later in this chapter) to develop an interval within which there is a defined probability (usually 95%) of the value of this measure being bounded. Notice that the 95% confidence interval is 7,083–7,825. This implies that for 95% of cases we are likely to find that the Years of Potential Life Lost Rate for Atlantic County is a number within the interval 7,083–7,825. This is an interval based on probabilities and gives us greater confidence (95% of cases) of a bound within which the true or population value is likely to lie.

The Z-score (Figure 4.1) provides a value in terms of standard deviations and is computed as the difference of the specific county value and the average for all counties in New Jersey and this difference is then divided by the standard deviation of the data. When the county value for Years of Potential Life Lost Rate is higher than the state average (as in the case of Atlantic County), the Z-score is positive; where this value is lower than the state average (as in the case of Bergen County), the Z-score is negative. Since the difference between the specific county value and the average for the state is divided by the standard deviation to get the Z-score, we can standardize the county values in relation to the state average and this provides a more meaningful comparison of the difference rather than just the absolute difference. The Z-score is a necessary first step in undertaking a Z-test to determine the statistical significance of the difference (see "Z-test" later in this chapter).

that in 95% of cases the population value of the measure is likely to be in this interval. Reporting these bounds in addition to the point estimate is increasingly becoming the norm. Thus, it is a good idea to understand how these bounds are computed.

The costs of collecting data from the entire population are usually prohibitive and thus we resort to a workaround to this by collecting information on a subset of the population or a sample. For instance, when we collect information on large demographic and health surveys, we sample the population in a country; if we survey patients from a hospital, we survey a sample of patients. Since the data thus collected are from only a sample and not the underlying population, we would like to test how estimates or measures from this sample data compare with population values of these estimates and measures. Based on probability of distributions, we assess, with varying degrees of certainty, our confidence in these estimates from the sample and how representative they are of the population. This process is aided by setting bounds on the data (confidence interval) and hypothesis testing.

For a detailed understanding of the theory behind setting bounds and hypothesis testing, refer to statistical texts (Kanji, 2009; Keller, 2006) and see Chapter 10, Sampling and Research Design Using Healthcare Data in Excel®, for a brief discussion of "Research Design" and "Sampling."

4.2 Setting Bounds on Data

Once sample data are collected, we establish bounds in relation to estimates from this sample within which we expect, with some level of certainty, the population value to be. In using trade-offs of the level of certainty, by convention we use 95% confidence intervals around the sample estimate within which we expect that 95% of the time, the population value will lie within this interval. Of course, we run a 5% chance that the population value may be outside this confidence interval. Confidence intervals are based on standard deviations representing the area under a normal curve. Here, 95% confidence intervals represent 1.96 times the standard error on either side of the normal curve while a 90% confidence interval represents 1.645 times the standard error. The trade-off here is that using a confidence interval less than 95% will lead to both a smaller confidence interval (1.645 times vs. 1.96 times the standard error) as well as a greater chance (10% vs. 5%) of the population value lying outside these bounds.

4.3 Sample and Population

A confidence interval has an upper and lower bound around the sample estimate. For instance, if we estimate a mean value from sample data, we can create bounds around this mean within which, 95% of the time, we expect the population value to lie.

For this example, we will use Dataset 3, the HCAHPS survey (see Box 4.2 for a brief description of HCAHPS surveys) conducted in Veterans Administration (VA) facilities (Centers for Medicare and Medicaid Services [CMS], 2016). Since the VA facilities are unique in terms of the patient demographics that they serve as well as the very insulated system (compared to other health facilities), the HCAHPS survey results for VA facilities are not included in the general HCAHPS survey reporting. This survey was conducted in 2017 and data are available from

123 of the 170 VA facilities. Data in this example are based on surveys completed by patients who were admitted to these VA facilities. The composite measures in this example are drawn from several questions on surveys completed by these patients. Let us focus on computing the bounds for this data.

BOX 4.2 HOSPITAL CONSUMER ASSESSMENT OF HEALTHCARE PROVIDERS AND SYSTEMS

Hospital X is a medium-sized hospital. As part of its customer experience system, the hospital encourages all patients to complete a brief customer experience survey using their smartphones or through available touchscreens. Data from these surveys are periodically summarized and shared at internal meetings to develop action steps that respond to the survey results.

Collecting customer experience is a laudable and worthy enterprise. However, each hospital is likely to have a different survey instrument and methodology for collecting and analyzing these surveys. The result is that there are as many different surveys as there are hospitals and no way to compare these results. In response to this dilemma, beginning in 2007-08, the CMS began requiring hospitals to complete a standardized Hospital Consumer Assessment of Healthcare Providers and Systems (HCAHPS) survey (CMS, n.d.). Now, there is a standardized survey instrument, a protocol for sampling and systematically collecting data from patients, training in conducting this survey, an analysis plan for the several composite measures based on the 29-item survey instrument, as well as adjustment for patients and mode of data collection in developing the star-ratings. In keeping with the times and the opioid crisis, minor adjustments in the survey items related to HCAHPS composite measure of pain have been proposed for 2019.

Currently, the HCAHPS survey reports are updated every quarter and the summary reports are based on the last four quarters of data collection. The latest summary results on the 10 composite measures in HCAHPS surveys (see Exhibit 4.1) provide state-specific results, including the number of hospitals per state and their response rates. The availability of state-specific results and the sample of hospitals facilitates comparison of these results across states (see "Hypothesis Testing" later in this chapter).

(continued)

EXHIBIT 4.1
SUMMARY OF HCAHPS SURVEY RESULTS (JAN.–DEC. 2017)

STATE	COMM. WITH NURSES	COMM. WITH DOCTORS	RESPONSIVENESS OF HOSPITAL STAFF	COMM. ABOUT MEDICINES	CLEANLINESS OF HOSP. ENV.	QUIETNESS OF HOSP. ENV.	DISCHARGE INFORMATION	CARE TRAN- SITION	HOSPITAL RATING	RECOMMEND THE HOSPITAL	PARTICI- PATING HOSPITALS*	SURVEY RESPONSE RATE*
AK	79	80	74	66	74	57	84	48	68	72	16	22%
AL	81	84	71	68	74	70	87	51	72	71	89	26%
AR	81	83	72	67	76	67	84	53	73	70	71	26%
AZ	78	77	67	64	74	56	86	51	70	70	75	29%
CA	76	77	63	63	72	52	85	49	69	70	327	23%
CO	80	81	72	67	77	63	88	56	75	75	70	27%
CT	80	80	65	62	74	55	87	52	71	73	30	27%
DC	71	76	53	58	64	55	83	45	62	62	8	23%
DE	81	80	69	66	73	57	88	54	72	71	7	24%

Source: From Hospital Consumer Assessment of Healthcare Providers and Systems. (2018, October 31). *Summary of HCAHPS survey results: January 2017 to December 2017 discharges.* Retrieved from https://www.hcahpsonline.org/globalassets/hcahps/summary-analyses/summary-results/2018_10_summary-_analysis_states_results.pdf

4.4 Measure and Variation

Consider the variable "Patients who understood their care." For this variable, we have the percentages from patient surveys for each of the 123 VA facilities. In the last cell in this column, we will first compute the average for this variable (Figure 4.2). Next, we need the standard error of this average in order to compute the bounds for our population value for patients who understood their care. The computation of standard error is a two-step process: first compute the standard deviation for this variable; and then divide the standard deviation by the square root of the sample size ($n = 123$) to get the standard error.

The formula for computing standard deviation in Excel has several variants to the general formula STDEV. The suffix "P" denotes that this formula is to be used for computing the standard deviation for data on the entire population. If we had data from all 170 VA medical facilities, we would use this formula. Since the suffix "S" denotes the use of formula for data from a sample (123 of the 170 VA facilities), we will go ahead and use "STDEV.S" to compute the standard deviation for the variable "Patients who understood their care."

Once the standard deviation is computed, we move on to compute the standard error of the mean. This is achieved by dividing the standard deviation by the square root of the sample size (123) in our example.

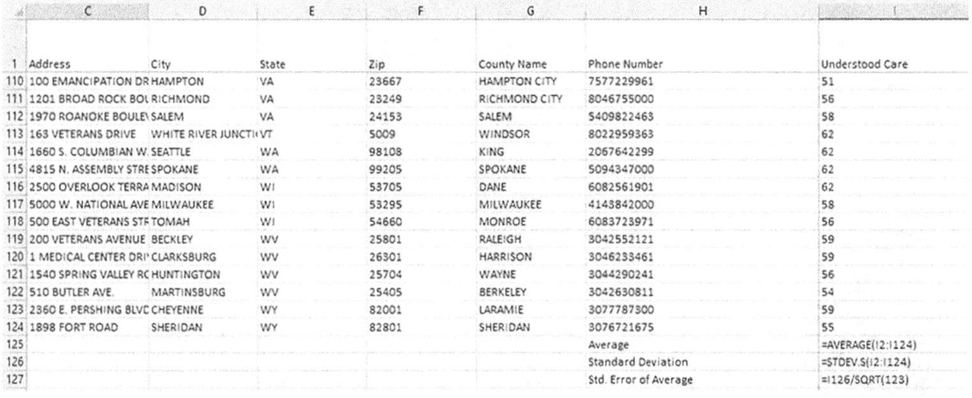

	C	D	E	F	G	H	I
1	Address	City	State	Zip	County Name	Phone Number	Understood Care
110	100 EMANCIPATION DR	HAMPTON	VA	23667	HAMPTON CITY	7577229961	51
111	1201 BROAD ROCK BOL	RICHMOND	VA	23249	RICHMOND CITY	8046755000	56
112	1970 ROANOKE BOULE\	SALEM	VA	24153	SALEM	5409822463	58
113	163 VETERANS DRIVE	WHITE RIVER JUNCTI	VT	5009	WINDSOR	8022959363	62
114	1660 S. COLUMBIAN W.	SEATTLE	WA	98108	KING	2067642299	62
115	4815 N. ASSEMBLY STRE	SPOKANE	WA	99205	SPOKANE	5094347000	62
116	2500 OVERLOOK TERRA	MADISON	WI	53705	DANE	6082561901	62
117	5000 W. NATIONAL AVE	MILWAUKEE	WI	53295	MILWAUKEE	4143842000	58
118	500 EAST VETERANS STF	TOMAH	WI	54660	MONROE	6083723971	56
119	200 VETERANS AVENUE	BECKLEY	WV	25801	RALEIGH	3042552121	59
120	1 MEDICAL CENTER DRI	CLARKSBURG	WV	26301	HARRISON	3046233461	59
121	1540 SPRING VALLEY RC	HUNTINGTON	WV	25704	WAYNE	3044290241	56
122	510 BUTLER AVE.	MARTINSBURG	WV	25405	BERKELEY	3042630811	54
123	2360 E. PERSHING BLVC	CHEYENNE	WY	82001	LARAMIE	3077787300	59
124	1898 FORT ROAD	SHERIDAN	WY	82801	SHERIDAN	3076721675	55
125						Average	=AVERAGE(I2:I124)
126						Standard Deviation	=STDEV.S(I2:I124)
127						Std. Error of Average	=I126/SQRT(123)

FIGURE 4.2 Computing average, standard deviation, and standard error of mean.

Tutorial video for Sections 4.4 and 4.5 is available by accessing the following url: https://connect.springerpub.com/content/book/978-0-8261-5028-8/chapter/ch11

4.5 Confidence Interval

The bounds also referred to as "confidence intervals" are computed as Mean ± 1.96*(Standard Error of Mean). In this formula, the factor 1.96 is related to the area under the normal curve and ensures that 95% of the area under the normal curve would be included within the lower and upper bounds. If we want the 90% confidence interval, the multiplication factor in the formula would be 1.645. As discussed in the earlier section ("Setting Bounds on Data") in this chapter, there is a trade-off in reducing the confidence level from 95% to 90%—tighter bounds (note the smaller multiplication factor) but a greater probability (10%) of the population value not being in the tighter bounds. Using the computations of average (mean) and standard error of the mean that we just undertook, we can compute the lower (Mean – 1.96*Standard Error of Mean) and upper bound (Mean + 1.96*Standard Error of Mean). In our example, the average is 55.42 and the standard error of the mean is 0.43 (Figure 4.3). Using the formula for the lower and upper bound, we get 54.58 and 56.26, respectively. This implies that 95% of the time we would expect the population mean for this variable to be within the confidence interval (54.58, 56.26). Something very striking about this confidence interval is clearly the tight bounds (54.58, 56.26). In addition to the confidence level, the tightness of the bounds is a function of the sample size and the population. Since our sample consists of over 70% of the population of VA medical facilities, it is no surprise that we have relatively tight confidence intervals for the population value of mean for "patients who understood their care." If our sample was much smaller, we would expect the confidence interval to be less tightly bound.

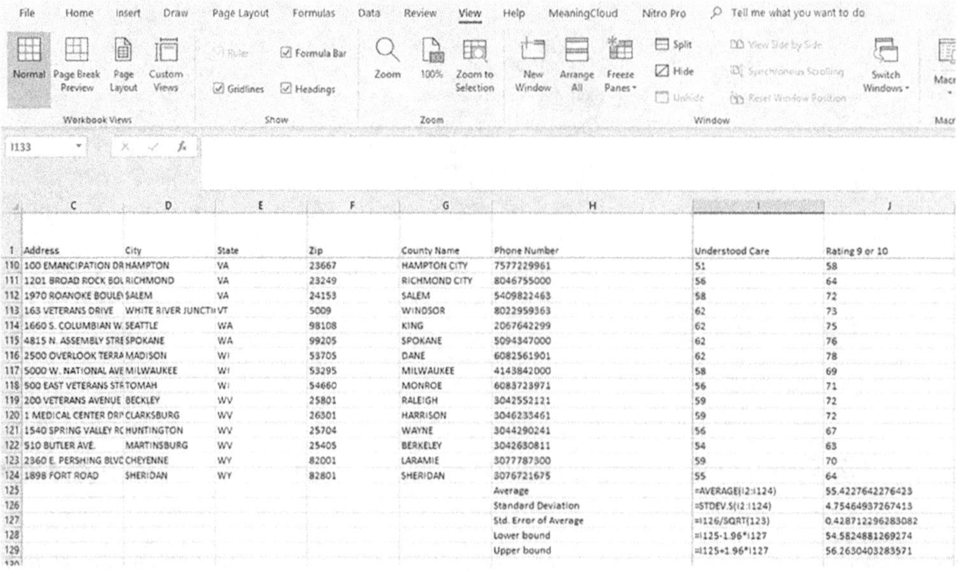

	C	D	E	F	G	H	I	J
1	Address	City	State	Zip	County Name	Phone Number	Understood Care	Rating 9 or 10
110	100 EMANCIPATION DR	HAMPTON	VA	23667	HAMPTON CITY	7577229961	51	58
111	1201 BROAD ROCK BOL	RICHMOND	VA	23249	RICHMOND CITY	8046755000	56	64
112	1970 ROANOKE BOULE\	SALEM	VA	24153	SALEM	5409822463	58	72
113	163 VETERANS DRIVE	WHITE RIVER JUNCTI	VT	5009	WINDSOR	8022959363	62	73
114	1660 S. COLUMBIAN W.	SEATTLE	WA	98108	KING	2067642299	62	75
115	4815 N. ASSEMBLY STRE	SPOKANE	WA	99205	SPOKANE	5094347000	62	76
116	2500 OVERLOOK TERRA	MADISON	WI	53705	DANE	6082561901	62	78
117	5000 W. NATIONAL AVE	MILWAUKEE	WI	53295	MILWAUKEE	4143842000	58	69
118	500 EAST VETERANS STR	TOMAH	WI	54660	MONROE	6083723971	56	71
119	200 VETERANS AVENUE	BECKLEY	WV	25801	RALEIGH	3042552121	59	72
120	1 MEDICAL CENTER DRI	CLARKSBURG	WV	26301	HARRISON	3046233461	59	72
121	1540 SPRING VALLEY RC	HUNTINGTON	WV	25704	WAYNE	3044290241	56	67
122	510 BUTLER AVE.	MARTINSBURG	WV	25405	BERKELEY	3042630811	54	63
123	2360 E. PERSHING BLVC	CHEYENNE	WY	82001	LARAMIE	3077787300	59	70
124	1898 FORT ROAD	SHERIDAN	WY	82801	SHERIDAN	3076721675	55	64
125						Average	=AVERAGE(I2:I124)	55.4227642276423
126						Standard Deviation	=STDEV.S(I2:I124)	4.75464937267413
127						Std. Error of Average	=I126/SQRT(123)	0.428712296283082
128						Lower bound	=I125-1.96*I127	54.5824881269274
129						Upper bound	=I125+1.96*I127	56.2630403283571

FIGURE 4.3 Computing confidence interval.

In computing the confidence interval that will bound our population value, we relied on using statistical functions in Excel. Within Excel, the use of the formula for confidence interval can cut down some of the computation that we undertook earlier. In order to use this formula for confidence interval, we need to clarify a few parts of the formula. This formula requires the alpha value, standard deviation of the sample mean, and the sample size (Figure 4.4). For 95% confidence interval, alpha is equal to (1 − 0.95 = 0.05). Once we input the required three arguments in this function, the confidence factor is computed. Mean ± this confidence factor gives us the lower and upper bound. In contrast to the earlier computation of the confidence interval, where we needed to additionally compute the standard error of the mean and then multiply it by 1.96 and then use this ± the mean to get the confidence interval, this appears more straightforward.

As an exercise, we can also use the formula for confidence interval to compute the 90% confidence interval. This formula requires the alpha value, standard deviation of the sample mean, and the sample size (Figure 4.4). For 90% confidence interval, alpha is equal to (1 − 0.90 = 0.10). Once we input the required three arguments in this function, the confidence factor is computed. Mean ± this confidence factor gives us the lower and upper bound. Based on this computation, the 90% confidence interval is (54.72, 56.13) while the 95% confidence interval is (54.58, 56.26). Notice that, as expected, there is the trade-off between the tightness of the bounds and the lower confidence level.

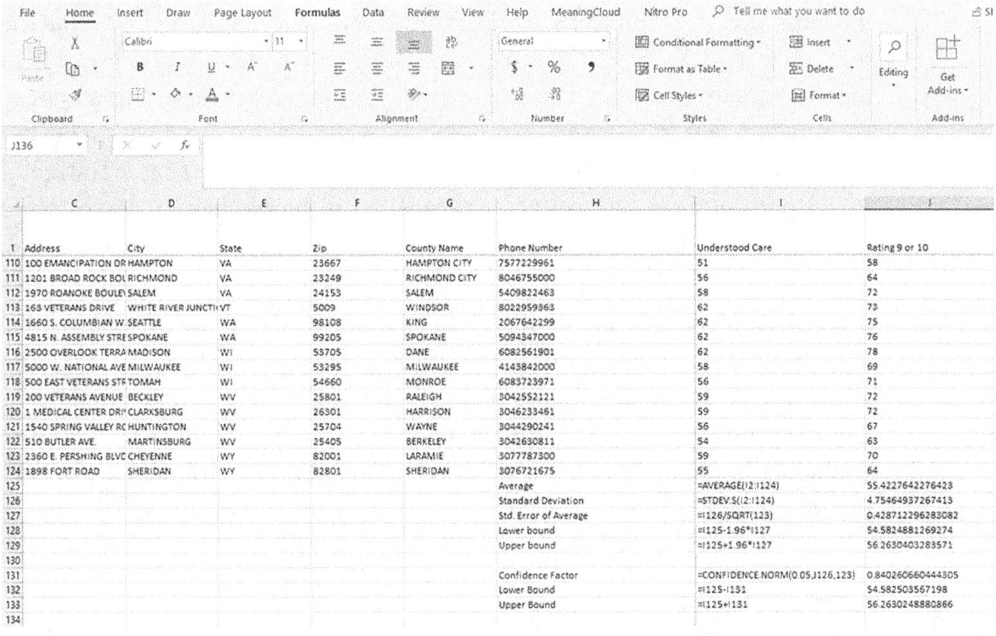

	C	D	E	F	G	H	I	J
1	Address	City	State	Zip	County Name	Phone Number	Understood Care	Rating 9 or 10
110	100 EMANCIPATION DR	HAMPTON	VA	23667	HAMPTON CITY	7577229961	51	58
111	1201 BROAD ROCK BOL	RICHMOND	VA	23249	RICHMOND CITY	8046755000	56	64
112	1970 ROANOKE BOULE\	SALEM	VA	24153	SALEM	5409822463	58	72
113	163 VETERANS DRIVE	WHITE RIVER JUNCTI	VT	5009	WINDSOR	8022959363	62	73
114	1660 S. COLUMBIAN W	SEATTLE	WA	98108	KING	2067642299	62	75
115	4815 N. ASSEMBLY STRE	SPOKANE	WA	99205	SPOKANE	5094347000	62	76
116	2500 OVERLOOK TERRA	MADISON	WI	53705	DANE	6082561901	62	78
117	5000 W. NATIONAL AVE	MILWAUKEE	WI	53295	MILWAUKEE	4143842000	58	69
118	500 EAST VETERANS STF	TOMAH	WI	54660	MONROE	6083723971	56	71
119	200 VETERANS AVENUE	BECKLEY	WV	25801	RALEIGH	3042552121	59	72
120	1 MEDICAL CENTER DRI	CLARKSBURG	WV	26301	HARRISON	3046233461	59	72
121	1540 SPRING VALLEY RC	HUNTINGTON	WV	25704	WAYNE	3044290241	56	67
122	510 BUTLER AVE.	MARTINSBURG	WV	25405	BERKELEY	3042630811	54	63
123	2360 E. PERSHING BLVC	CHEYENNE	WY	82001	LARAMIE	3077787300	59	70
124	1898 FORT ROAD	SHERIDAN	WY	82801	SHERIDAN	3076721675	55	64
125						Average	=AVERAGE(I2:I124)	55.4227642276423
126						Standard Deviation	=STDEV.S(I2:I124)	4.75464937267413
127						Std. Error of Average	=I126/SQRT(123)	0.428712296283082
128						Lower bound	=I125-1.96*I127	54.5824881269274
129						Upper bound	=I125+1.96*I127	56.2630403283571
130								
131						Confidence Factor	=CONFIDENCE.NORM(0.05,J126,123)	0.840260660444305
132						Lower Bound	=I125-I131	54.582503567198
133						Upper Bound	=I125+I131	56.2630248880866
134								

FIGURE 4.4 Using CONFIDENCE function.

4.6 Hypothesis Testing

In setting the bounds, we have already introduced the idea of sample estimates and population values. We always use the sample estimates to create the bounds within which we have some confidence (usually 95%) that the population values would be. Thus, we expect 95% of the time that the population value would be within the bounds of this confidence interval.

This setup leads us directly to the notion of hypothesis testing. Our hypothesis is stated in terms of population values (not sample estimates). The hypothesis is stated as both the original hypothesis (H_0) and the alternate hypothesis (H_1 or H_A). Stating our hypothesis in these two forms facilitates testing as well as rejecting or failing to reject these hypotheses. There are two overarching approaches to set up the alternate hypothesis: one is that the population value is not a certain value (not equal to); the other is that the population value is greater than or less than a certain value. We will use the example on HCAHPS survey from VA Medical Facilities to set up our alternate hypothesis using these two overarching approaches.

4.6.1 Alternate Hypothesis Not Equal to Population Value

In this approach, we could state our hypothesis as:

H_0: The population mean for patients who understood their care is 50%.

H_A: The population mean for patients who understood their care is not 50%.

Note that the hypotheses are developed independent of the confidence intervals or setting bounds to the sample estimate and usually set at the midpoint of all possible values (Quirk, 2016). Of course, it is also possible to identify other population values based on other sources of data. This allows us to test whether it is possible for our sample to come from a population having a population mean of 50% of patients who understood their care. Testing of this hypothesis is undertaken by ascertaining if the population mean in the hypothesis is within the confidence interval or bounds of the sample estimate. Since the confidence interval is (54.58, 56.26), we are 95% confident that our population mean of 50% does not fall within these bounds. Based on this confidence interval, we reject the original hypothesis and instead accept the alternate hypothesis that the population mean is not 50%. Since there is never 100% certainty in accepting or rejecting these hypotheses, research literature would also state this as failure to accept (for rejecting) and failure to reject (for accepting).

Tutorial video for Section 4.6 is available by accessing the following url: https://connect .springerpub.com/content/book/978-0-8261-5028-8/chapter/ch11

4.6.2 Alternate Hypothesis Greater Than (or Less Than) Population Value

In this approach, we could state our hypothesis as:

H_0: The population mean for patients who understood their care is 50%.

H_A: The population mean for patients who understood their care is greater than 50%.

This allows us to test whether it is possible for our sample to come from a population having a population mean of greater than 50% of patients who understood their care. Testing of this hypothesis is undertaken by ascertaining if the population mean in the hypothesis is in the confidence interval or bounds of the sample estimate. Since the confidence interval is (54.58, 56.26), we are 95% confident that our population mean of 50% does not fall within these bounds. Based on this confidence interval, we reject the original hypothesis and instead accept the alternate hypothesis that the population mean is greater than 50%.

4.7 Z-Test

▶ Thus far we have discussed hypothesis testing of a hypothesized population value in relation to confidence intervals. Excel also includes a function that performs the Z-test to assess null and alternate hypotheses based on the population mean (Kanji, 2009). There are assumptions underlying the use of the Z-test, the most important of which is a sample size is conservatively greater than 60. The Z-test in Excel gives us the probability of Z. Before we conduct the Z-test in Excel, we give a few points of clarification about the probability distribution that will be used for interpreting the results of this test.

The Z-test in Excel returns the probability of Z in the distribution assuming a one-tailed test. The one-tailed test is akin to testing our alternate hypothesis stated as greater than (or less than) the population value in the null hypothesis. This formula for the Z-test in Excel is adapted to also return the probability of Z in the distribution assuming a two-tailed test. Here, the two-tailed test is the same as testing our alternate hypothesis stated as not equal to the population value. If the probability in either the one-tailed or two-tailed Z-test is less than 0.05, we reject the null hypothesis and accept the alternate hypothesis. Let us work through the same example that we used for the confidence interval to see how the Z-test would be done in Excel and the results interpreted.

4.7.1 One-tailed Z-test

If we state our hypotheses as:

H_0: The population mean for patients who understood their care is 50%.

▶ Tutorial video for Section 4.7 is available by accessing the following url: https://connect .springerpub.com/content/book/978-0-8261-5028-8/chapter/ch11

H_A: The population mean for patients who understood their care is greater than 50%.

This is the setup for a one-tailed Z-test in Excel. Since we are undertaking a Z-test using the variable "Patients who understood their care," go to an empty cell in the worksheet containing this variable and enter the function "=Z.Test" and press "enter" (Figure 4.5). The formula then prompts you to enter "array"—this is the entire column of data for our variable. Separate the next argument in this formula with a comma and the formula then prompts you to enter "x"—this is the hypothesized population value (50) that we need to enter. Beyond the "array" and "x," there is "[sigma]." Sigma refers to the population standard deviation if it is known from other data. In this case, we do have the sample standard deviation, not the population standard deviation. However, this is not an issue as anytime an argument in a function is enclosed in square brackets ([ ]) it is optional. If we have the population value we include it; if we don't have it—as in this case—we skip over it, close the parentheses, and press "enter" to get the results of the formula (Figure 4.5).

Based on this one-tailed Z-test, the probability of Z is 5.668...E-37. The probability is a very, very small number—a decimal followed by 36 zeros and 5668. Since the probability of Z is clearly less than 0.05, we reject the null hypothesis and accept the alternate hypothesis that the population mean for patients who understood their care is greater than 50%.

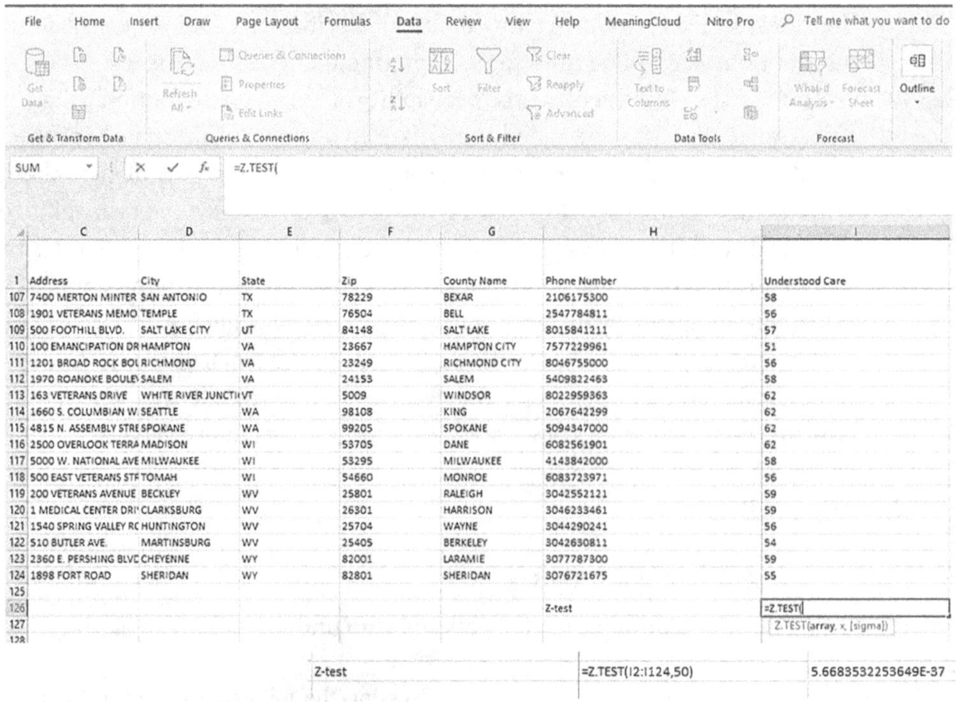

FIGURE 4.5 One-tailed Z-test in Excel.

4.7.2 Two-tailed Z-test

Now, if our hypotheses are:

H_0: The population mean for patients who understood their care is 50%.

H_A: The population mean for patients who understood their care is not 50%.

This is the setup for a two-tailed Z-test in Excel. Since we are undertaking a Z-test using the variable "Patients who understood their care," go to an empty cell in the worksheet containing this variable. In this empty cell, we will not enter the function for the Z-test—since that computes the one-tailed probability and we need the two-tailed probability. In the empty cell, we will use the function for the Z-test and modify it to provide the two-tailed probability. Enter in this empty cell "=2*MIN(Z.test(Array,x),1-Z.test(Array,x))." As before, in this formula "array" is the entire column of data for our variable and "x" is hypothesized population value (50) that we are testing (Figure 4.6). The output of this function gives us the probability of Z for a two-tailed distribution—as before, it is a very, very small number—a decimal followed by 35 zeros and 1133. Since the probability of Z is clearly less than 0.05, we reject the null hypothesis and accept the alternate hypothesis that the population mean for patients who understood their care is not 50%.

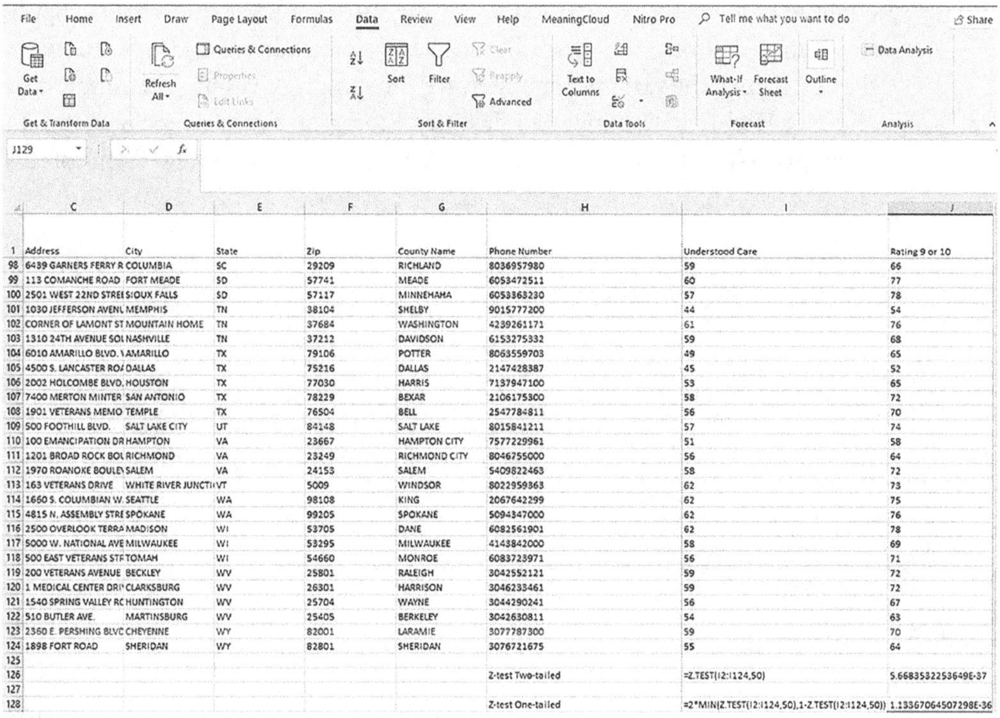

FIGURE 4.6 Two-tailed Z-test in Excel.

4.8 Comparing Two Samples Using the Z-Test

Consider the variable "Patients who understood their care." For this variable, we have the percentages from patient surveys for each of the 123 VA facilities. A Z-test for this data is useful to assess if there are differences in this variable for two categories in this dataset. Categories, if available, could be size of facility, age of facility, or some other category that might be relevant to the variable that we are testing. Since the dataset does not contain any relevant category variable, let us include a category that identifies the VA facility as being "Highly Recommended." Here, Highly Recommended is based on the percentage of patients who recommended the hospital using the third quartile as the cutoff to create a "Highly Recommended" and a "Not Highly Recommended" category. This is achieved by using an IF statement (Figure 4.7) to categorize as HI (for Highly Recommended) and LO (for Not Highly Recommended). Next, we can either work on this data in the same sheet or, just to focus on this analysis, copy the two columns containing the Highly Recommended data and the categories (HI and LO) that were just created and paste them into a new worksheet. In this new worksheet, select the two columns of data and sort using the HI and LO column. After sorting, copy and paste in a column labeled HI all the data that corresponds to the HI category. Next, copy the LO category data and paste into the adjacent column labeled LO (Figure 4.8).

In order to test if the means for patients who understood their care is different based on whether the patients received care in a VA facility that is Highly Recommended or not, we need to undertake one additional step—compute the variance of the variable separately for the sample of Highly Recommended and Not Highly Recommended facilities. Compute the variance by going to an empty cell and using the function "=VAR.S." There are several forms of this

| N2 | | | f_x | =IF(M2>=75,"HI","LO") | | | | | | |

	C	D	E	F	G	H	J	K	L	M	N
								Doc	Nurse		
					County		Room Quiet at	Communicati	Communicati	Recommend	
1	Address	City	State	Zip	Name	Phone Number	Night	on	on	Hospital	
2	700 SOUTH	BIRMINGH	AL	35233	JEFFERSON	2059334515	61	80	72	62	LO
3	215 PERRY	MONTGOI	AL	36109	MONTGOI	3342604100	71	76	73	60	LO
4	1100 N. CO	FAYETTEVI	AR	72703	WASHING	4794445058	52	77	77	77	HI
5	4300 WEST	LITTLE ROC	AR	72205	PULASKI	5012571000	51	80	73	66	LO
6	650 E. INDI/	PHOENIX	AZ	85012	MARICOP/	6022226444	44	73	72	58	LO
7	500 HIGHW	PRESCOTT	AZ	86313	YAVAPAI	9284454860	63	79	81	74	LO
8	3601 SOUTI	TUCSON	AZ	85723	PIMA	5206291821	50	70	75	72	LO
9	2615 E. CLII	FRESNO	CA	93703	FRESNO	5592285338	37	78	66	59	LO
10	11201 BENT	LOMA LINI	CA	92357	SAN BERN/	9098257084	36	75	67	69	LO
11	5901 E. SEV	LONG BEA(	CA	90822	LOS ANGEI	5628268000	43	78	75	66	LO
12	11301 WILS	LOS ANGEI	CA	90073	LOS ANGEI	3104783711	42	74	67	58	LO
13	10535 HOSI	MATHER	CA	95655	SACRAMEI	8003828387	47	80	77	73	LO
14	3801 MIRAI	PALO ALTC	CA	94304	SANTA CLA	6508583939	54	82	79	84	HI

FIGURE 4.7 Creating category.

Tutorial video for Section 4.8 is available by accessing the following url: https://connect.springerpub.com/content/book/978-0-8261-5028-8/chapter/ch11

	A	B	C	D	E	F	G
	Recommend						
1	Hospital	HI or LO			HI	LO	
2	77	HI			77	62	
3	84	HI			84	60	
4	75	HI			75	66	
5	75	HI			75	58	
6	76	HI			76	74	
7	88	HI			88	72	
8	86	HI			86	59	
9	78	HI			78	69	
10	77	HI			77	66	
11	75	HI			75	58	
12	82	HI			82	73	
13	84	HI			84	66	
14	76	HI			76	59	
15	75	HI			75	73	
16	76	HI			76	69	
17	80	HI			80	53	
18	76	HI			76	70	
19	85	HI			85	67	
20	82	HI			82	67	
21	78	HI			78	71	
22	81	HI			81	67	
23	77	HI			77	62	
24	82	HI			82	74	
25	77	HI			77	74	
26	78	HI			78	63	
27	75	HI			75	64	
28	76	HI			76	64	
29	80	HI			80	70	
30	76	HI			76	65	
31	80	HI			80	73	
32	77	HI			77	62	
33	77	HI			77	72	
34	78	HI			78	64	

FIGURE 4.8 Focusing on HI and LO data.

function that are available in Excel. The "S" suffix indicates its use in computing variance for a sample. We will compute the variance twice—once for the sample of VA facilities in Highly Recommended facilities and once for Not Highly Recommended facilities (Figure 4.9).

Once the variance is computed, we can use the Analysis ToolPak option (see Chapter 1, Introduction to Healthcare Data and the Role of Excel®), to undertake a Z-test. Click on "Data" in the toolbar. In the ribbon that opens up, at the extreme right of the screen is the "Data Analysis" option (Figure 4.10). Click on

	A	B	C	D	E	F
1	Recommend Hospital	HI or LO			HI	LO
86	72	LO				70
87	68	LO				72
88	71	LO				68
89	68	LO				73
90	57	LO				68
91	71	LO				
92	56	LO	Variance (HI)	=VAR.S(E2:E35)	12.6497326203209	
93	69	LO				
94	72	LO	Variance (LO)	=VAR.S(F2:F90)		37.326353421859
95	63	LO				

A2 · fx 77

FIGURE 4.9 Computing variance.

"Data Analysis" and within the menu that opens, scroll down to choose "Z-test." In the Z-test menu that is revealed, we identify the variable 1 (HI) and variable 2 (LO) samples for patients who understood their care by clicking on the "up arrow" next to each of these variables and then selecting the relevant range of data for these two samples for the data on patients who understood their care. Next, type "0" for hypothesized mean difference for our null hypothesis of no difference in mean values of patients who understood their care for the sample of VA facilities in coastal and inland states. For this hypothesized

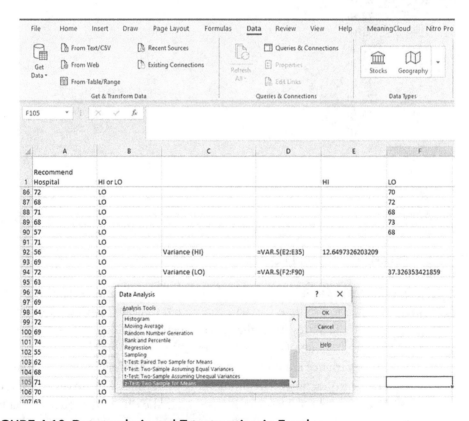

FIGURE 4.10 Data analysis and Z-test option in Excel.

mean difference, we can also include values other than zero that we would like to test. For the "Variable variance known" we need to enter the variances for the Highly Recommended (HI) and Not Highly Recommended (LO) samples that we computed—making sure to enter the value for "Highly Recommended" for Variable 1 and "Not Highly Recommended" for Variable 2 (see Figure 4.11). Since our sample data include labels in the patients who understood their care data column for "HI" and "LO," make sure that this is checked. This box will be checked any time the data for the two categories (Highly Recommended and Not Highly Recommended) appear in separate columns. The options for data output allow you to control where the output is going to be placed. It is easiest to let the output be placed in a separate worksheet.

Click on the new worksheet where your output for the Z-test is placed (Figure 4.12). You will have to resize the columns to make sure that you can see the entire output. In the output, in the first four rows, there is a summary of the two samples—Highly Recommended (Variable 1) and Not

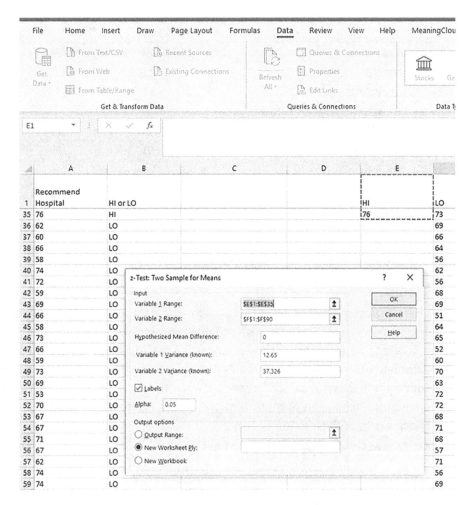

FIGURE 4.11 Z-test for two samples.

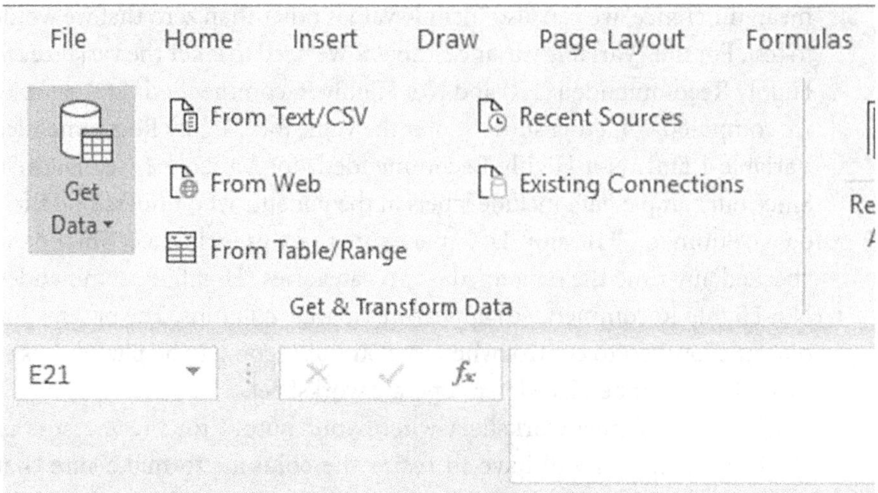

	A	B	C
1	z-Test: Two Sample for Means		
2			
3		*HI*	*LO*
4	Mean	78.67647059	66.05617978
5	Known Variance	12.65	37.326
6	Observations	34	89
7	Hypothesized Mean Difference	0	
8	z	14.18590508	
9	P(Z<=z) one-tail	0	
10	z Critical one-tail	1.644853627	
11	P(Z<=z) two-tail	0	
12	z Critical two-tail	1.959963985	
13			

FIGURE 4.12 Z-test output for two samples.

Highly Recommended (Variable 2)—for the data on patients who understood their care. The first row provides the means for the two samples, the second row includes the variance that we inputted, the third has the number of observations for each sample, while the fourth row includes our hypothesized mean difference between the two samples of zero. In the remaining rows, the output for the Z-test is given. This output tests two alternate hypotheses:

First hypothesis tested (one-tailed test)

H_O: There is no difference in mean values of samples of Highly Recommended and Not Highly Recommended VA facilities on patients who understood their care.

H_{A1}: The mean value of Highly Recommended VA facilities on patients who understood their care is greater than the mean value in Not Highly Recommended VA facilities.

Second Hypothesis tested (two-tailed test)

H_O: There is no difference in mean values of samples of Highly Recommended and Not Highly Recommended VA facilities on patients who understood their care.

H_{A2}: The mean values of samples of Highly Recommended and Not Highly Recommended VA facilities on patients who understood their care is not identical.

We continue with reviewing the results in our output of the Z-test. There is a "z" value that is computed based on the summary in the first four rows of our output. This "z" value is then tested based on whether we are testing the first hypothesis (one-tailed) or second hypothesis (two-tailed). The conclusions of the Z-test are based on either the probability of the Z-test or a comparison of the "z" value to the relevant critical value. For the first hypothesis, the probability of z-value (p(Z(<=z) one tail) is 0.00%. Anytime the probability of z is less than 0.05%, we fail to accept (in other words, we reject) the null hypothesis. Alternatively, we can compare the "z" value with the relevant critical "z" value. Our z value of 14.186 is greater than the critical z value (one tail) of 1.64. Since our z value is greater than the critical z value, we fail to accept the null hypothesis. "Failing to accept" is the same as "rejecting" our null hypothesis of no difference in mean values of patients who understood their care in Highly Recommended and Not Highly Recommended VA facilities.

For the second hypothesis (two-tailed), the probability of z value (P(Z<=z) two tail) is also 0.00%. Since this probability is less than 0.05%, we fail to accept the null hypothesis. Since the "z" value is greater than the critical z value for two-tail, we fail to accept the null hypothesis. This conclusion can be stated alternatively as rejecting (failing to accept) the null hypothesis. Notice that whether we use the probability or comparison to critical z value, our conclusions will be identical. In our example, for both alternate hypotheses, based on probabilities and critical z values, we fail to accept (or in other words, we reject) the null hypothesis of no difference in mean values for patients who understood their care in Highly Recommended and Not Highly Recommended VA facilities.

4.9 Competency Development

In Box 4.1, we were introduced to the County Health Rankings and how these rankings acknowledge uncertainty in computation of estimates and allow for this by reporting the computed estimates, the confidence interval, as well as the z-scores. The practice of reporting the confidence interval and/or the z-values whenever estimates are computed from datasets allows for the inherent uncertainty in these computations rather than the misplaced preciseness of a point estimate. Through these practices, we have access to probabilistic estimates and a range of certainty where, in 95% of cases, our estimate is likely to lie. In addition, z-values standardize the generated estimates and thus make it easier to compare different estimates. These practices engender the competency domain of problem-solving.

Healthcare is replete with several examples that are ripe for comparison. In Box 4.2, we are introduced to the HCAHPS. These surveys allow hospitals to compare different points of service delivery as well as to compare their scores to those of their peers or competitors. As a precursor to this comparison, we are introduced to the computation in Excel of z-scores through the standard error (standard deviation divided by the square root of the sample size). The standard error of the mean is then used to further compute bounds or confidence intervals within which we usually expect the population value 95% of the time. Either computed thus or through the available Excel formula for confidence interval, we get these bounds that then allow for testing hypotheses about comparison of sample and population values. In addition to using confidence intervals for hypothesis testing, Excel includes, through the Analysis ToolPak add-in, a routine to complete a Z-test. The Z-test allows us to choose and assess two categories of variables and systematically compare them on outcomes (when the sample size is greater than 30). The thinking through of hypotheses, including whether to use a one-sided or two-sided option, builds applications from the competency domain of critical thinking. The testing of these hypotheses, through computation of confidence intervals or the Z-test in Excel, strengthens the competency domain in performance management.

The focus of professional education is the development of competencies such that students develop skills in the application of a variety of tools and skills. In this chapter, emphasis is on the development of critical thinking, analytical or problem-solving (Commission on Accreditation of Healthcare Management Education, 2018), as well as performance management competencies.

4.10 Summary

Within the healthcare setting, we have access to several datasets from public and institutional settings. In this chapter, we are introduced to County Health Rankings as well as HCAHPS. Since these and other data are based on sample data, not the entire population, there is a certain lack of certainty associated with point estimates based on these datasets. Using bounded 95% confidence intervals, we can gain certainty that the population value of any measure would be bounded within the confidence interval.

Z-scores are used to standardize measures in relation to their average values by dividing the difference between a point estimate and its average value by the standard deviation. These Z-scores are the precursors to Z-tests used for testing a variety of hypotheses as well as testing the equality of two samples (greater than 30).

4.11 Discussion Questions

4.11.1 What causes uncertainty in estimates from sampled data? How would you increase certainty in estimates from sampled data?

4.11.2 How would you test the mean of sampled data?

4.11.3 You have the means on smoking rates from two counties served by your hospital. How would you test to see if there is truly a difference in the two means?

4.12 Practice Problems

All datasets required for the practice problems are available for download at http://connect.springerpub.com/content/book/978-0-8261-5028-8.

4.12.1 As the analyst for the health advocacy group, you have just presented data on premature deaths and poor or fair health from Dataset 5. For these two fields compute:

  a. Average value
  b. Standard deviation
  c. Standard error of the mean
  d. 90% Confidence interval around the mean

Next, scroll to column MG in your dataset—percent of population that is female. How would you test a hypothesis about the underlying population of females being 50%?

  e. State your null and alternate hypotheses.
  f. Undertake computation to test this hypothesis.
  g. Report the results and interpretation of any tests that you undertake.

4.12.2 The VA is concerned about the experience of customers at VA facilities. In 2017, HCAHPS surveys were completed in a large sample of VA facilities nationwide. These data are available in Dataset 3. Senior management is convinced that Communication With Nurses is the problem. Use this dataset to better understand the variable Communication With Nurses by computing:

  a. Average value
  b. Standard deviation
  c. Standard error of the mean
  d. 95% Confidence interval around the mean

Tutorial videos provided for Practice Problems 4.12.1—4.12.7 can be accessed by accessing the following url: https://connect.springerpub.com/content/book/978-0-8261-5028-8/chapter/ch11

You hypothesize that Communication With Nurses varies with Patient Recommendation of Hospital. Categorize facilities as Highly Recommended if 75% or more of patients recommend the facility; else the facility is Not Highly Recommended. How would you test a hypothesis about the equality of Communication With Nurses across Highly Recommended and Not Highly Recommended VA facilities?

    e. State your null and alternate hypotheses.

    f. Undertake computation to test this hypothesis.

    g. Report the results and interpretation of any tests that you undertake.

4.12.3 The VA is concerned about the experience of customers at VA facilities. In 2017, HCAHPS surveys were completed in a large sample of VA facilities nationwide. These data are available in Dataset 3. Senior management is convinced that Communication With Doctors is the problem. Use this dataset to better understand the variable Communication With Doctors by computing:

    a. Average value

    b. Standard deviation

    c. Standard error of the mean

    d. 95% Confidence interval around the mean

Consider the variables in the dataset. By which variable (choose only one) would you hypothesize that Communication With Doctors varies? How would you test a hypothesis about the equality of Communication With Doctors across this chosen variable?

    e. Justify your choice of variable.

    f. State your null and alternate hypotheses.

    g. Undertake computation to test this hypothesis.

    h. Report the results and interpretation of any tests that you undertake.

4.12.4 The VA is concerned about the experience of customers at VA facilities. In 2017, HCAHPS surveys were completed in a large sample of VA facilities nationwide. This data is available in Dataset 3. Senior management is convinced that Cleanliness of Hospital Environment is the problem. Use this dataset to better understand the variable Cleanliness of Hospital Environment by computing:

    a. Average value

    b. Standard deviation

    c. Standard error of the mean

    d. 95% Confidence interval around the mean

You hypothesize that Cleanliness of Hospital Environment varies with Patient Rating of Hospital. Categorize facilities as Highly Rated if 75% or more of patients rated the facility highly; else the facility is Not Highly Rated. How would you test a hypothesis about the equality of Cleanliness of Hospital Environment across Highly Rated and Not Highly Rated VA facilities?

    e. State your null and alternate hypotheses.

    f. Undertake computation to test this hypothesis.

    g. Report the results and interpretation of any tests that you undertake.

4.12.5 Data summary for October 2018 for HCAHPS surveys nationwide is available. These data are available in Dataset 10. As a policy analyst, you would like to see what the experience of patients with Cleanliness of Hospital Environment is. Use this dataset to better understand the variable Cleanliness of Hospital Environment by computing:

    a. Average value

    b. Standard deviation

    c. Standard error of the mean

    d. 95% Confidence interval around the mean.

You hypothesize that Cleanliness of Hospital Environment varies with Patient Rating of Hospital. Categorize facilities as Highly Rated if 75% or more of patients rated the facility highly; else the facility is Not Highly Rated. How would you test a hypothesis about the equality of Cleanliness of Hospital Environment across Highly Rated and Not Highly Rated facilities?

    e. State your null and alternate hypotheses.

    f. Undertake computation to test this hypothesis.

    g. Report the results and interpretation of any tests that you undertake.

4.12.6 Data on health insurance coverage by state as of December 2016 are available in Dataset 9. As an analyst with the healthcare insurance industry, you would like to see what the effect of Medicaid expansion on health insurance coverage has been. Use this dataset to better understand the variable "Uninsured rate 2015" by computing:

    a. Average value

    b. Standard deviation

    c. Standard error of the mean

    d. 95% Confidence interval around the mean

You hypothesize that with Medicaid expansion, uninsured rates will go down. How would you test a hypothesis about Medicaid expansion and uninsured rates?

    e. State your null and alternate hypotheses.

    f. Undertake computation to test this hypothesis.

    g. Report the results and interpretation of any tests that you undertake.

4.12.7 Data on health insurance coverage by state as of December 2016 are available in Dataset 9. As an analyst with the healthcare insurance industry, you would like to see what the effect of Medicaid expansion on employer-provided health insurance coverage has been. Use this dataset to better understand the variable 'Employer coverage 2015' by computing:

a. Average value

b. Standard deviation

c. Standard error of the mean

d. 95% Confidence interval around the mean

You hypothesize that with Medicaid expansion, employer-provided coverage will go down. How would you test a hypothesis about Medicaid expansion and employer-provided coverage?

e. State your null and alternate hypotheses.

f. Undertake computation to test this hypothesis.

g. Report the results and interpretation of any tests that you undertake.

See Chapter 11, Video Tutorials and Answers to Practice Problems Using Healthcare Datasets in Excel®, for video answers to the practice problems.

References

Centers for Medicare and Medicaid Services. (n.d.). About Hospital Compare data. Retrieved from https://www.medicare.gov/hospitalcompare/Data/Overview.html

Centers for Medicare and Medicaid Services. (2016, October 19). Veterans Health Administration hospital performance data. Retrieved from https://www.cms.gov/Medicare/Quality-Initiatives-Patient-Assessment-Instruments/HospitalQualityInits/VA-Data.html

Commission on Accreditation of Healthcare Management Education. (2018). *CAHME eligibility requirements*. Retrieved from https://www.cahme.org/files/accreditation/FALL2017_CAHME_CRITERIA_FOR_ACCREDITATION_2018_06_01.pdf

County Health Rankings and Roadmaps. (n.d.). Explore health rankings: Rankings data and documentation. Retrieved from http://www.countyhealthrankings.org/explore-health-rankings/rankings-data-documentation

Hospital Consumer Assessment of Healthcare Providers and Systems. (2018, October 31). *Summary of HCAHPS survey results: January 2017 to December 2017 discharges*. Retrieved from https://www.hcahpsonline.org/globalassets/hcahps/summary-analyses/summary-results/2018_10_summary-_analysis_states_results.pdf

Kanji, G. K. (2009). *100 statistical tests* (3rd ed., reprinted). London, United Kingdom: Sage Publications.

Keller, D. K. (2006). *The tao of statistics: A path to understanding (with no math)*. Thousand Oaks, CA: Sage Publications.

Quirk, T. J. (2016). *Excel 2016 for health services management statistics: A guide to solving practical problems*. New York, NY: Springer.

5

TESTING AND COMPARING MEANS OF HEALTHCARE DATASETS USING EXCEL®

LEARNING OBJECTIVES

- Appreciate the use of *t*-test for drawing inferences from small samples
- Use descriptive statistics to assess data distribution assumptions for using *t*-test
- Understand when to use different versions of the *t*-test
- Interpret results from hypothesis testing

In this chapter, we will use the t-test in Excel to compare the means of two groups of data. Variations of the t-test allow us to make different assumptions about the underlying population including unequal variances and paired samples to have greater confidence in inferences based on small samples. In this chapter, the competency domains of critical thinking, problem-solving, and performance management are emphasized.

5.1 *t*-Test

Thanks to William Sealy Gossett a.k.a "Student" (see Box 5.1), one of the most commonly used and robust statistical tests is the *t*-test. Broadly, the *t*-test assesses the significance of the difference in average or mean value of data for two groups. It is robust because this test can be undertaken even for smaller samples (<60). This is done for a variety of comparisons of different samples or categories of data (Kanji, 2009; Quirk, 2016).

Throughout the chapter supplemental content is available for the datasets and tutorial videos. Video availability is denoted with an icon. To gain access to these items, please visit the following urls:

Datasets: https://connect.springerpub.com/content/book/978-0-8261-5028-8

⊙ Tutorial Videos: https://connect.springerpub.com/content/book/978-0-8261-5028-8/chapter/ch11

BOX 5.1 A TOAST TO THE *T*-TEST

In 1908, William Sealy Gossett developed the *t*-test (Encyclopedia Britannica, n.d.) and testing small samples (<30) to make inferences about estimates from these small samples was never the same again. William was neither a mathematician nor a statistician—he happened to work at a brewery in England (Kopf, n.d.). His supervisor and he were tasked with testing samples of hops used for brewing beer to ensure adherence to quality standards. At that time, making inferences was based on very large samples. Rather than wait for the large samples of hops to materialize and make inferences, his supervisor had small samples (<15) from which he wanted to make inferences about the quality of the hops. He turned to Gossett to take this work forward and to come up with a probabilistic distribution that would give confidence on inferences drawn from these small samples. By a process of trial and error and through repeated draws of samples of hops, in time, Gossett developed a distribution and sought help from mathematicians to confirm and formalize his work culminating in the *t*-distribution and its associated probabilities for estimates from small samples.

The story does not end here. He wanted to publicize his work, but his brewery did not want his work to be published as their competitors would then start using Gossett's work to fine-tune their approach to quality. As a compromise, the brewery agreed to let Gossett publish under an alias. Gossett chose "Student" as his alias and so the *t*-distribution is also known as the "Student *t*-distribution" (Student, n.d.).

As health professionals, there are several comparisons in which we are interested. Following the Tripe Aim framework (Institute for Healthcare Improvement, 2012) to guide decision-making, we will be looking to make decisions affecting the patient experience, health of populations, as well as per capita cost. These decisions could lead to questions such as:

- Are there differences in an intervention and control group?
- Are there differences in patient experiences in two departments of a hospital?
- Do death rates for men and women in a state vary significantly over time?
- Do the per capita costs for a hospital vary significantly from state and national averages for similar hospitals?

Making these decisions requires enormous amounts of data. However, with the *t*-test and its robustness, even with small samples, there is greater confidence in using smaller datasets to make these decisions. To see how this is possible, let us use data in a variety of contexts to see how the *t*-test is useful for decision-making.

5.2 Assumptions for the *t*-Test

Since we are dealing with smaller samples, it is important to consider the assumptions that need to be met, to choose which of the three broad variants of the *t*-test (British Medical Journal, n.d.; Kanji, 2009) should be used, and to have confidence in the results. Three assumptions for the *t*-test are:

a. Normal distribution

b. Equal standard deviation

c. Independent observations

The independent observation is to ensure that data are not collected repeatedly from the same sample. By using descriptive statistics in Excel (see Chapter 3, Identifying, Categorizing, and Presenting Healthcare Data Using Excel®), we can see if our data is approximately normally distributed as well as how different the standard deviations are. Approximately normal data will have skewness and kurtosis values between −2 and +2 and the mean and median will be very similar. If the standard deviation of the two groups differs by a factor of 2, we could say that the two groups have unequal variances. Should these measures not give a clear picture of the approximate normal distribution of data, more elaborate procedures in Excel (e.g., Chi-Square Goodness-of-Fit) and other specialized statistical software that can aid a more complete assessment of normality are recommended.

5.3 Example for *t*-Test

For this example, we will use Dataset 3, the Hospital Consumer Assessment of Healthcare Providers and Systems (HCAHPS) survey conducted in Veterans Administration (VA) facilities. This survey was conducted in 2017 and data is available from 123 of the 170 VA facilities. Data in this example are based on surveys completed by patients who were admitted to these VA facilities. The composite measures in this example are drawn from several questions on surveys completed by these patients (see Box 4.2 for a brief overview of the HCAHPS survey and data).

Consider the variable "Patients who understood their care." For this variable, we have the percentages from patient surveys for each of the 123 VA facilities. A *t*-test for these data is useful to assess if there are differences in this variable for two categories in the dataset. Categories, if available, could be size of facility, age of facility, or some other category that might be relevant to the variable that we are testing. Because the dataset does not contain any relevant category variable, let us see if there are differences in the mean percentages of patients

---

Tutorial video for Section 5.3 is available by accessing the following url: https://connect.springerpub.com/content/book/978-0-8261-5028-8/chapter/ch11

who understood their care if these patients went on highly rated VA facilities versus if they did not. Here "highly rated" can be defined based on percentile and we can choose the 75th percentile for "rating of 9 or 10" to divide our data into two groups—highly rated (above 75th percentile) and not highly rated (below 75th percentile). We can then formalize our testable hypotheses as:

H_0 (null hypothesis): There is no difference in mean value of patients who understood care in VA facilities that are highly rated or not highly rated.

H_A (alternate hypothesis): The mean value of patients who understood care is higher in VA facilities that are highly rated than if they are not highly rated.

In order to undertake this comparison, first we need to find the threshold for dividing the data into two groups, that is, the 75th percentile. We go to the data and scroll down to the bottom of the column containing data "rating of 9 or 10" (see Figure 5.1). Here we enter the formula for computing percentile "=percentile.exc." This formula prompts us to identify the data array (cells where our entire data on this variable are found) and then enter the percentile as a decimal value (0.75). Through this we determine that our 75th percentile is at the data value of 74.

Next, select the entire data—all rows and columns—and click on "Data" on the toolbar and choose "Sort" (Figure 5.2). In the Sort Panel that opens, make sure to choose the variable "rating of 9 or 10" for the first "sort by" column and the variable "understood care" for the next "then by" column. If additional levels of sorting are visible, make sure to delete these levels using the "delete level" tab at the top of the Sort Panel.

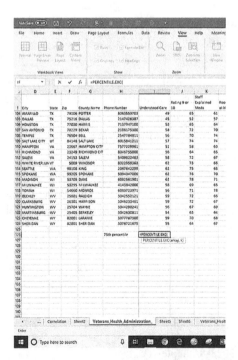
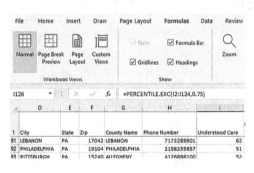

FIGURE 5.1   Categorizing data into groups.

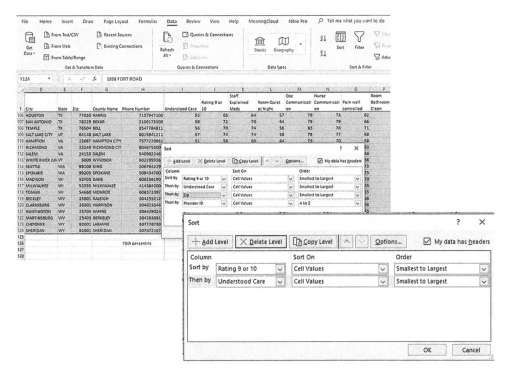

FIGURE 5.2 Sorting data for groups.

Before we proceed to the actual *t*-test, we need to run descriptive statistics (Chapter 3, Identifying, Categorizing, and Presenting Healthcare Data Using Excel®, section on "Descriptive Statistics") on our two groups to see how the assumptions of the *t*-test are met and what variant of the *t*-test we should use. Note that these descriptive statistics will be for the variable "understood care" and not "rating of 9 or 10." This is because the rating variable is used only to categorize our data into two groups.

The output for descriptive statistics for each of these two groups, Highly Rated and Not Highly Rated (Figure 5.3), show that the means and medians for the two groups are very similar and the skewness and kurtosis are close to zero—indicating an approximately normal distribution. Because the standard deviations of the two groups are approximately similar, we conclude that the variances of the two groups are equal. The data are also independent as the samples are not repeated in our dataset.

Now we are ready to undertake a test of comparison using the *t*-test. The *t*-test is invoked through the toolbar by clicking on "Data" and then choosing the "Data Analysis" option that opens at the far right. Clicking on "Data Analysis" leads to several statistical procedures and tests that can be done in Excel. Because we are interested in the *t*-test, we scroll through the list till we come to *t*-test (Figure 5.4).

Through the Data Analysis tab, it is possible to undertake three variants of the *t*-test (Kanji, 2009) in Excel (Quirk, 2016). The variants use different assumptions about the underlying data to complete these tests.

Not Highly Rated			Highly Rated	
Column1			*Column1*	
Mean	53.90625		Mean	60.8148148
Standard Error	0.393220544		Standard Erroi	0.69805802
Median	54		Median	61
Mode	56		Mode	61
Standard Deviation	3.852758752		Standard Devi	3.6272159
Sample Variance	14.84375		Sample Variar	13.1566952
Kurtosis	0.090512759		Kurtosis	-0.0317445
Skewness	-0.002690786		Skewness	0.32311188
Range	20		Range	15
Minimum	44		Minimum	54
Maximum	64		Maximum	69
Sum	5175		Sum	1642
Count	96		Count	27

FIGURE 5.3 Descriptive statistics for groups.

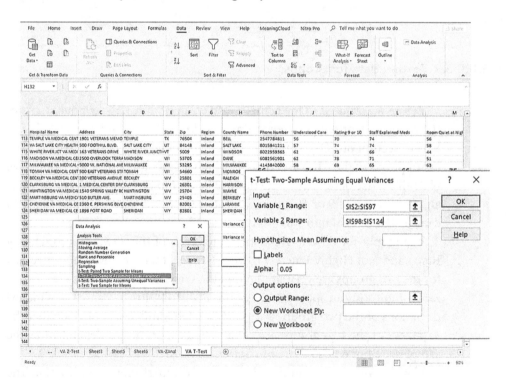

FIGURE 5.4 *t*-Test using Analysis ToolPak in Excel.

5.3.1 *t*-Test Two-Sample Mean Assuming Equal Variance

This *t*-test is done when we are interested in comparing samples that are differentiated by a category (highly rated and not highly rated facilities in our example) under the assumption that the populations underlying these two categories have equal variance for the variable (patients who understood their care).

5.3.2 *t*-Test Two-Sample Mean Assuming Unequal Variance

This *t*-test is done when we are interested in comparing samples that are differentiated by a category (highly rated and not highly rated facilities in our example) under the assumption that the populations underlying these two categories have unequal variance for the variable (patients who understood their care). Variance of the two categories would be considered unequal if the standard deviation of the two categories differs by a factor of 2.

5.3.3 *t*-Test Paired Two-Sample Mean

This *t*-test is done when we are interested in the results of a pre- and posttest that is undertaken with the same sample. Because we have "pairs" of data from the same sample, we can undertake the "Paired Two-Sample Mean" *t*-test in this situation.

5.4 *t*-Test Two-Sample Mean Assuming Equal Variance

Because our descriptive statistics helped us to ascertain the approximate normal distribution of our data and that there is equal variance in the two groups (highly rated and not highly rated VA facilities), we choose "*t*-test: Two-Sample Assuming Equal Variance." In the panel that opens, we identify the data array for Variable 1 as the variable "patients who understood care" for VA facilities that are not highly rated, that is, "star rating 9 or 10" value less than 75. Variable 2 is similarly identified for VA facilities that are highly rated, that is, "star rating 9 or 10" value 75 or higher. Because our null hypothesis is that there is no difference, we can leave the "Hypothesized Mean Difference" blank. For the groups for which we did not create any labels—because the data are in one column—we therefore will not check the box for "Labels" and we make no change to the "Alpha" of 0.05 since we are testing at the standard 95% (1–0.95 = 0.05) level of significance. Finally, depending on where we want our output of this *t*-test to go, we can check the appropriate box for output options.

The resulting output for this *t*-test is in Figure 5.5. Here Variable 1 is our group of VA facilities that are not highly rated and Variable 2 is the group of VA facilities that are highly rated. We see the mean of our data and the number of observations—just to confirm from our earlier descriptive statistics (see Figure 5.3) that we have included the correct range of data on "patients who understood their care" for each of these groups. Our null hypothesis of mean difference of zero appears in this output. Finally, we see our probability of this *t*-stat for one-tail—because our alternate hypothesis is that the mean value for

Tutorial video for Section 5.4 is available by accessing the following url: https://connect .springerpub.com/content/book/978-0-8261-5028-8/chapter/ch11

t-Test: Two-Sample Assuming Equal Variances

	Variable 1	Variable 2
Mean	53.90625	60.8148148
Variance	14.84375	13.1566952
Observations	96	27
Pooled Variance	14.4812423	
Hypothesized Mean Difference	0	
df	121	
t Stat	-8.33393039	
P(T<=t) one-tail	7.1265E-14	
t Critical one-tail	1.65754432	
P(T<=t) two-tail	1.4253E-13	
t Critical two-tail	1.97976376	

FIGURE 5.5 *t*-Test: Two-sample assuming equal variance.

"patients who understood their care" is higher in VA facilities that are highly rated. This probability is a very small number, that is, 13 zeros after the decimal. Because this probability is less that 0.05 (our chosen level of significance), we fail to accept our null hypothesis and thus accept the alternate hypothesis that the mean value for "patients who understood their care" is higher in VA facilities that are highly rated than in VA facilities that are not highly rated.

5.5 *t*-Test Two-Sample Mean Assuming Unequal Variance

The National Center for Health Statistics (NCHS) is a Center within the Centers for Disease Control and Prevention (CDC). NCHS is better known for the collection of vital statistics from the state-based vital statistics registries. It has a very active website (www.cdc.gov/nchs/) for access to several public use databases as well as visualizations. One visualization of the death rates and life expectancy (Figure 5.6) in the United States is for the period 1900 to 2015. In this figure, the death rates have been declining and the life expectancy has been increasing—except for the anomaly in 1918 to 1919—presumably on account of World War I. Data such as these might prompt a question as to how mortality varies between males and females.

In the NCHS data file, Dataset 11, we have data on deaths among males and females by state for this period. For purposes of understanding differences

Tutorial video for Section 5.5 is available by accessing the following url: https://connect.springerpub.com/content/book/978-0-8261-5028-8/chapter/ch11

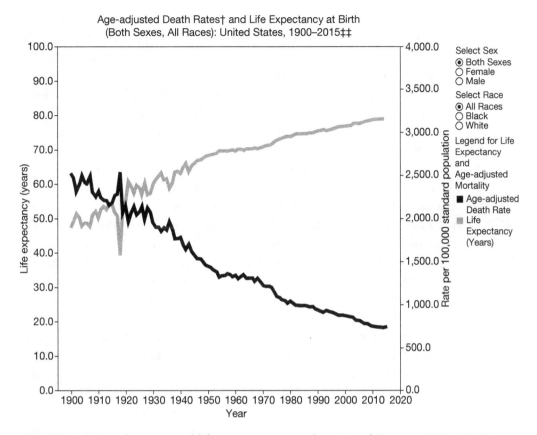

FIGURE 5.6 **Death rates and life expectancy in the United States (1900–2017).**

NOTE: †Age-adjusted death rates (deaths per 100,000) after 1998 are calculated based on the 2000 U.S. standard population. Populations used for computing death rates for 2011 to 2015 are postcensal estimates based on the 2010 census, estimated as of July 1, 2010. Rates for census years are based on populations enumerated in the corresponding censuses. Rates for noncensus years between 2000 and 2010 are revised using updated intercensal population estimates and may differ from rates previously published. Data on age-adjusted death rates prior to 1999 are taken from historical data. ‡‡ Life expectancy data are available up to 2014. Due to changes in categories of race used in publications, data are not available for the Black population consistently before 1968, and not at all before 1960. More information on historical data on age-adjusted death rates is available at www.cdc.gov/nchs/nvss/mortality/hist293.htm.

SOURCE: Bastian, B., Tejada Vera, B., Arias, E., et al. (2019). Mortality trends in the United States, 1900–2017. National Center for Health Statistics. Retrieved from https://www.cdc.gov/nchs/data-visualization/mortality-trends

among males and females, for now we will focus the analysis on the first state in this list—Alabama. The hypothesis that we are trying to test is:

H_0: There is no difference in number of deaths in males and females in Alabama for the period 1999 to 2016.

H_A: The number of deaths in males in Alabama during the period 1999 to 2016 is higher than in females.

To test this hypothesis in our small sample of 18 data points each for males and females, we can consider the *t*-test. However, we need to ascertain the underlying assumptions about the data distribution by running descriptive statistics (as described in Figure 5.3 earlier).

Figure 5.7 contains the descriptive statistics separately for deaths in males and females in Alabama during 1999 to 2016. The mean and median for females are very similar and the skewness and kurtosis are within the range of −2 to +2 to approximate a normal distribution. For males, the mean and median are somewhat distinct, while the skewness and kurtosis are within tolerable range to approximate a normal distribution. Next, we consider the standard deviation of the two distributions. The standard deviation for males is 1.8 times that for females. This implies that the variance of the two samples is unequal and we should use the *t*-test that allows for unequal variance.

This *t*-test is very similar to the *t*-test assuming equal variance (mentioned previously). The only difference is the assumption about the underlying data and the variance therein. Here we assume that the two samples have unequal variance. Using this assumption of unequal variance, we proceed as before to access through the "Data Analysis" tab, the *t*-test assuming unequal variance.

As in the *t*-test assuming equal variance (mentioned previously), we input the required information in the window that opens (Figure 5.8). The resulting output for *t*-test assuming unequal variance provides a summary of the data for Variable 1 (females) and Variable 2 (males), which we use to confirm that we have the correct data array for this *t*-test—the means for males and females as well as the number of observations are as obtained in the output for descriptive statistics. This is a one-tailed *t*-test as our alternate hypothesis is the number of deaths in males in Alabama during the period 1999 to 2016 is

Female		Male	
Mean	23897.7778	Mean	23926.056
Standard Error	191.706297	Standard Error	344.57416
Median	23872	Median	23571
Mode	#N/A	Mode	#N/A
Standard Deviation	813.340935	Standard Deviation	1461.9043
Sample Variance	661523.477	Sample Variance	2137164.3
Kurtosis	0.02876809	Kurtosis	-0.453643
Skewness	0.49964936	Skewness	0.7400448
Range	3015	Range	4661
Minimum	22603	Minimum	22187
Maximum	25618	Maximum	26848
Sum	430160	Sum	430669
Count	18	Count	18

FIGURE 5.7 Descriptive statistics for male and female deaths in Alabama (1999–2016).

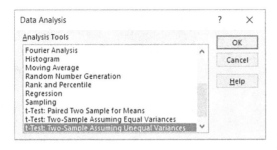

t-Test: Two-Sample Assuming Unequal Variances

	Femqle	Males
Mean	23897.8	23926.1
Variance	661523	2137164
Observations	18	18
Hypothesized M	0	
df	27	
t Stat	-0.07171	
P(T<=t) one-tail	0.47168	
t Critical one-ta	1.70329	
P(T<=t) two-tail	0.94336	
t Critical two-ta	2.05183	

FIGURE 5.8 *t*-test: Two-sample assuming unequal variance.

higher than in females. We confirm, through the high *t*-statistic and the very low probability (decimal followed by 25 zeros) of this *t*-statistic, the one-tailed probability that we fail to accept (reject) the null hypothesis of no difference in mean deaths among males and females in Alabama during 1999 to 2016. Instead, we accept (fail to reject) the alternate hypothesis that mean deaths among males in Alabama during 1999 to 2016 is higher than among females.

5.6 *t*-Test Paired Two-Sample Mean

In situations where there are pre- and postintervention measures on the same sample, we have a classic case of a paired sample. For instance, in a hypothetical case, if we were to implement an intervention in VA medical facilities to boost scores for the variable patients who understood their care, the *t*-test Paired Two-Sample Mean is used to determine if the intervention changed the scores pre and post the intervention. To test this, there are hypothetical data on 30 facilities pre- and postintervention in the included worksheet (Figure 5.9). For this data, we have the following hypotheses:

H_O: There is no difference in mean scores for patients who understood care pre- and postintervention.

H_A: Mean scores for patients who understood care postintervention are greater than preintervention.

Tutorial video for Section 5.6 is available by accessing the following url: https://connect .springerpub.com/content/book/978-0-8261-5028-8/chapter/ch11

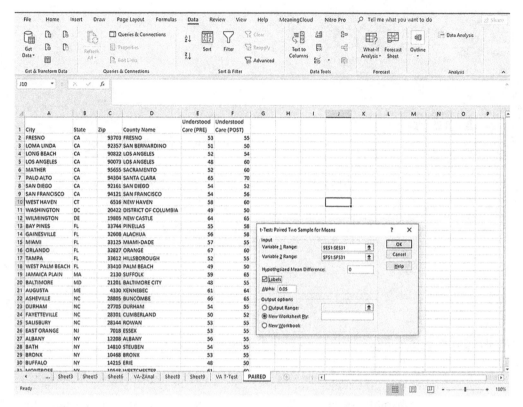

FIGURE 5.9 *t*-Test for paired two-sample mean.

Using the procedure described in the earlier section, we use the "Data Analysis" tab to access the procedures and tests and navigate to "*t*-test: Paired Two-Sample Mean" (Figure 5.10). In the window that opens, we need to identify the ranges for Variable 1 (pre) and Variable 2 (post). Do this by clicking on the "up arrow" next to each of these variables and selecting the entire range of data corresponding to each of these variables. As per our hypothesis, we include that the hypothesized mean difference between pre and post is zero. Note that because we have data in two separate columns (pre and post), we can check the box next to "label." This will identify to Excel that the first row in the range does not include data. Finally, the default option for the output to appear in a new worksheet is left as is.

Accessing the data output from the new worksheet, we see that the first five rows of output summarize our data and our hypothesis that we are testing. The *t* statistic or value is −3.027. Since our hypothesis is stated as a one-tail test (alternate hypothesis is postintervention is greater than pre-), we look at the probability of *p* value for one-tail test ($P(T \leq t)$ one tail). This probability is 0.257% which is below 5% so we fail to accept (reject) the null hypothesis of no difference in mean scores pre- and postintervention. Thus, we accept the alternate hypothesis that the mean scores for patients who understood their care post the intervention are greater than preintervention.

	File	Home	Insert	Draw	Page Layout	Formulas	Data	Review

Get Data ▾	Refresh All ▾	☐ Queries & Connections Properties Edit Links	A↓ Z↓	Sort	Filter

Get & Transform Data | Queries & Connections | Sort & Fi

B18 | : | × | ✓ | fx |

◢	A	B	C	
1	t-Test: Paired Two Sample for Means			
2				
3		*Understood Care (PRE)*	*Understood Care (POST)*	
4	Mean	55.06666667	56.96666667	
5	Variance	29.51264368	25.96436782	
6	Observations	30	30	
7	Pearson Correlation	0.788603164		
8	Hypothesized Mean Difference	0		
9	df	29		
10	t Stat	-3.027304978		
11	P(T<=t) one-tail	0.002568197		
12	t Critical one-tail	1.699127027		
13	P(T<=t) two-tail	0.005136394		
14	t Critical two-tail	2.045229642		
15				

FIGURE 5.10 Data output from *t*-test paired two-sample mean.

5.7 Competency Development

In a perfect world, we have large samples with which to work and have confidence in the results and tests based on these large samples. However, it is very difficult to have these conditions met in real life. What do we do then? As described in Box 5.1, we seek inspiration from the work of an old-time brewery worker, who was trying to make a call on quality based on small samples of hops—the work that eventually led to the *t*-distribution and *t*-test that is well-suited for small samples (n <60). In healthcare, the *t*-test is applied to test for statistical differences in small samples for several comparisons or hypotheses. These comparisons and hypotheses themselves are developed based on frameworks such as the Triple Aim. Thus, in developing testable hypotheses, we are exercising the competency domains of critical thinking and problem-solving.

Before undertaking the *t*-test, we need to make sure that the three key assumptions for the *t*-test—normal distribution, equal standard deviation, and independent observations—are met through using the descriptive statistics routine in Excel. Once this hurdle is crossed, and we have assessed how the assumptions are met, we are then ready to choose which of the three versions of the *t*-test—equal variance, unequal variance, or paired two-sample mean—to apply. Once the test is completed, the results need to be interpreted prior to decision-making. Assessing the assumptions as well as determining which of the three versions of the *t*-test to apply and interpreting the results, leads to application of the competency domains of problem-solving and performance management.

In this chapter, understanding the data distribution assumptions and their implications for choosing the correct variant of the *t*-test focus on competency domain of critical thinking. While, applying the correct *t*-test to small samples and interpreting the results focuses on the competency domains of performance management and problem-solving.

5.8 Summary

The t-*test is very ably suited for working with small samples and still having confidence in inferences drawn from these small samples. Key assumptions for using the* t-*test include normality of data distribution, variance, and independent samples. Within Excel, descriptive statistics help us to assess if the underlying data distribution is approximately normal. Depending on the equality of variance in groups of data, we can then determine which version of the* t-*test to use.* T-*test gives us greater confidence in hypothesis testing from small samples and interpreting results for decision-making in healthcare.*

5.9 Discussion Questions

5.9.1 What are the assumptions that need to be met for using the *t*-test?

5.9.2 How would you test the assumptions for using the *t*-test?

5.9.3 Does it make a difference as to which of the three versions of the *t*-test you use? Why or why not?

5.10 Practice Problems

(▶)   All datasets required for the practice problems are available for download at http://connect.springerpub.com/content/book/978-0-8261-5028-8.

5.10.1 You work at a policy think tank and are excited to get summary data on HCAHPS surveys nationwide. This data were generated in October 2018 and are available in Dataset 10. You are interested in assessing if

---

(▶) Tutorial videos provided for Practice Problems 5.10.1—5.10.8 can be accessed by accessing the following url: https://connect.springerpub.com/content/book/978-0-8261-5028-8/chapter/ch11

there is a significant difference in Communication With Doctors by the variable "rating." In order to test this difference:

a. Use a cutoff value of 80th percentile to assign a hospital as "Highly Rated" and "Not Highly Rated" below that cutoff.

b. Determine if the assumptions for t-test are met.

c. State your null and alternate hypothesis.

d. If the assumptions are met, proceed with undertaking the t-test twice—once assuming equal variance and once assuming unequal variance.

e. Which of these t-tests is appropriate for your data? Why?

f. Interpret the results of the t-test. What recommendations would you make based on this t-test?

5.10.2 In the dataset on HCAHPS survey at VA facilities (Dataset 3), create a category to separate VA facilities into "High" or "Low" recommendation for this facility. This category is based on the field "Recommend Hospital" and uses the median value of "Recommend" determining if the recommendation is high or low. Use this categorization to test if there is a difference in mean value of the variable "Understood Care."

a. Test the assumptions for using a t-test.

b. State your null and alternate hypotheses.

c. What test would you use?

d. Undertake the test and report your test statistics as well as interpretation.

5.10.3 Next, use the categorization of "high" and "low" recommendation (see 5.10.2) to test if there is a difference in mean value of the variable "Doctor Communication."

a. Test the assumptions for using a t-test.

b. State your null and alternate hypotheses.

c. What test would you use?

d. Undertake the test and report your test statistics as well as interpretation.

5.10.4 The Alabama Health Commissioner is very concerned about the health status and outcome in counties in Alabama. She has just received data on health of the counties in Dataset 7. She reaches out to you to figure out if there is any difference in counties with high age-adjusted mortality on the Motor Vehicle (MV) Mortality Rate. Use the dataset to do the following:

a. Develop criteria to assign counties as high age-adjusted mortality and those that are not high age-adjusted mortality.

b. What test will you use to assess if there is a difference in counties with high age-adjusted mortality and MV mortality rate?

    c. Test to see if the assumptions of the test are met.

    d. Run the test and interpret the results for the Health Commissioner.

5.10.5 The Alabama Health Commissioner is very concerned about the health status and outcome in counties in Alabama. She has data on health of the counties in Dataset 7. She reaches out to you to figure out if there is any difference in counties with high age-adjusted mortality and the percentage of uninsured adults. Use the dataset to do the following:

    a. Develop criteria to assign counties as high age-adjusted mortality and those that are not high age-adjusted mortality.

    b. What test will you use to assess if there is a difference in counties with high age-adjusted mortality and the percentage of uninsured adults?

    c. Test to see if the assumptions of the test are met.

    d. Run the test and interpret the results for the Health Commissioner.

5.10.6 The Alabama Health Commissioner is still very concerned about the health status and outcome in counties in Alabama. She has data on health of the counties in Dataset 7. She reaches out to you to figure out if there is any difference in counties with high age-adjusted mortality on the healthcare costs. Use the dataset to do the following:

    a. Develop criteria to assign counties as high age-adjusted mortality and those that are not high age-adjusted mortality.

    b. What test will you use to assess if there is a difference in counties with high age-adjusted mortality and healthcare costs?

    c. Test to see if the assumptions of the test are met.

    d. Run the test and interpret the results for the Health Commissioner.

5.10.7 As part of the ongoing discussions about impacts of healthcare reform and the role of public funding, federal level policy makers would like some idea of these impacts, especially as they relate to private sector coverage. Use Dataset 9 to analyze if a state having expanded Medicaid coverage has any effect on "Total with private coverage." Use the dataset to do the following:

    a. What test will you use to assess if there is a difference in states that expanded Medicaid coverage and private coverage in the state?

    b. Test to see if the assumptions of the test are met.

    c. Run the test and interpret the results for federal policy makers.

5.10.8 As part of the ongoing discussions about healthcare reform and insurance coverage, federal level policy makers would like some idea of preliminary impacts, especially as they relate to children gaining coverage by staying on their parents' plan. Use Dataset 9 to analyze if "Individuals who gained coverage by staying on their parents' plan" has any effect on the "People gaining coverage 2010-15." Use the dataset to do the following:

a. Develop criteria to assign "Individuals who gained coverage by staying on their parents' plan" as "high gain" and "low gain." Create a new variable that has these codes for high gain and low gain.

b. What test will you use to assess if there is a difference in states that had high or low gain for "Individuals who gained coverage by staying on their parents' plan' and 'People gaining coverage 2010 to 2015"?

c. Test to see if the assumptions of the test are met.

d. Run the test and interpret the results for federal policy makers.

See Chapter 11, Video Tutorials and Answers to Practice Problems Using Healthcare Datasets in Excel®, for video answers to the practice problems.

▪ References

Bastian, B., Tejada Vera, B., Arias, E., et al. (2019). Mortality trends in the United States, 1900–2017. National Center for Health Statistics. Retrieved from https://www.cdc.gov/nchs/data-visualization/mortality-trends

British Medical Journal. (n.d.). 7. The t tests. Retrieved from https://www.bmj.com/about-bmj/resources-readers/publications/statistics-square-one/7-t-tests

Encyclopedia Britannica. (n.d.). Student's t-test. Retrieved from https://www.britannica.com/science/Students-t-test

Institute for Healthcare Improvement. (2012). The IHI Triple Aim. Retrieved from http://www.ihi.org:80/Engage/Initiatives/TripleAim/Pages/default.aspx

Kanji, G. K. (2009). *100 statistical tests* (3rd ed., reprinted). London, UK: Sage Publications.

Kopf, D. (n.d.). The Guinness brewer who revolutionized statistics. *Priceonomics.* Retrieved from http://priceonomics.com/the-guinness-brewer-who-revolutionized-statistics

Quirk, T. J. (2016). *Excel 2016 for health services management statistics: A guide to solving practical problems.* New York: Springer.

Student. (n.d.). *The probable error of the mean.* Retrieved from https://www.york.ac.uk/depts/maths/histstat/student.pdf

6

CHECKING PATTERNS IN HEALTHCARE DATA USING SCATTERPLOTS, CORRELATIONS, AND REGRESSIONS IN EXCEL®

LEARNING OBJECTIVES

- Hypothesize relationships based on theory and expectations
- Explore relationships in pairs of variables using a scatterplot
- Describe how relationships between variables are used for healthcare decision-making
- Know how to undertake a correlation
- Learn to interpret correlations
- Understand the use of regressions in developing models of relationships among variables
- Interpret results from regression output
- Develop predictions based on regression equations
- Appreciate multicollinearity in multiple regression
- Impute missing values based on predictions from multiple regression models

In this chapter, we use scatterplots, correlations, and regressions in Excel to understand the relationship and patterns in data. The use of predictions from multiple regression to impute missing values is also considered. In this chapter, the competency domains of critical thinking, performance management, and problem-solving are emphasized.

Throughout the chapter supplemental content is available for the datasets and tutorial videos. Video availability is denoted with an icon. To gain access to these items, please visit the following urls:

Datasets: https://connect.springerpub.com/content/book/978-0-8261-5028-8

⊙ Tutorial Videos: https://connect.springerpub.com/content/book/978-0-8261-5028-8/chapter/ch11

BOX 6.1 CORRELATION OF HEALTHCARE COST, COVERAGE, AND ACCESS COMPONENTS

In 2012, PDA Inc and The Cecil B. Sheps Center for Health Services Research, University of North Carolina (UNC) at Chapel Hill submitted their commissioned report to the Appalachian Regional Commission (ARC). This report (Lane et al., 2012) undertook research into disparity in healthcare resources, coverage, and the cost of providing health services in 1,070 counties across the 13 Appalachian states. To do this, the two research agencies developed a county-level Healthcare Cost Coverage and Access (HCCA) Index. As part of the development of this Index, these agencies assessed several common health status measures and how they relate to the different components of the HCCA Index. One example of this is from Table 19 in this report (see Exhibit 6.1).

In the table in Exhibit 6.1, these agencies are investigating how Years of Potential Life Lost (YPPL) below 75 years of age relates to the HCCA Index as well as its components. The Index draws upon related dimensions of access to health professionals and facilities, health insurance coverage, and costs of healthcare. Further, in reflecting a social determinants framework, the relation of the HCCA Index with proportion of disability in the community as well as ARC's Economic Distress Index (EDI) was also explored, the idea here being that the Index should have a relationship to health outcomes as well as social determinants. To assess how the HCCA Index and its components relate to Years of Potential Life Lost as well as disability and economic distress, these agencies modified the measurement of the measures in this table to ensure that the results are easily interpretable. Details of these modifications can be found in the appendices to this report. Next, before applying this HCCA Index to the ARC counties, the agencies used available county-level data on these variables from all 3,110 counties in the United States.

- YPLL_75: Years of potential life lost under age 75 per 100,000 population, averaged over 2005 to 2007 and expressed as a percentile

- Disabled: Ratio of the number of disabled persons on Medicare (Supplementary Medical Insurance [SMI] and Hospital Insurance [HI]) to the estimated population for the same year (2007), expressed as a percentile

- ARC_EDI: ARC Economic Distress Index value rank (1 = Best; 3,110 = Worst)

- HCCA: Healthcare Cost, Coverage and Access Index, expressed as a percentile (1 = Best; 100 = Worst)

(continued)

EXHIBIT 6.1

CORRELATIONS BETWEEN HEALTH STATUS, ECONOMIC DISTRESS, AND PROPOSED HCCA COMPONENTS FOR ALL COUNTIES IN THE UNITED STATES.

VARIABLE	M (SD)	COMMUNITY HEALTH STATUS		ECONOMIC DISTRESS	PROPOSED INDEX AND COMPONENTS			
		YPLL_75	DISABLED	EDI	HCCA	HCRA	HIC	HCC
YPLL_75	49.5 (28.9)	1.000	.669	.669	.490	.288	.284	.465
Disabled	50.5 (28.9)	—	1.000	.672	.275	.183	-.031[NS]	.426
EDI	1552.0 (895.9)	—	—	1.000	.487	.360	.257	.424
HCCA	50.5 (28.9)	—	—	—	1.000	.710	.702	.703
HCRA	50.5 (28.9)	—	—	—	—	1.000	.264	.254
HIC	50.5 (28.9)	—	—	—	—	—	1.000	.244
HCC	50.5 (28.9)	—	—	—	—	—	—	1.000

EDI, economic distress index; HCCA, healthcare cost, coverage, and access; HCRA, healthcare resource availability; HIC, health insurance coverage; HCC, healthcare cost.

Note: Numbers of counties employed in the above correlations range from 3,008 to 3,110, depending on availability of YPLL_75 estimates for the counties. Estimates for YPLL_75 were missing in 95 cases, and judged to be unreliable in an additional 196 cases. All correlations are significant at the $p < .01$ level, except for those marked "NS."

Source: Lane, N. M., Lutz, A. Y., Baker, K., Konrad, T. R., Ricketts, T. R., Randolph, R., . . . Beadles, C. A. (2012). *Health care costs and access disparities in Appalachia* [Research report]. Retrieved from https://www.arc.gov/assets/research_reports/HealthCareCostsandAccessDisparitiesinAppalachia.pdf

(continued)

> ## BOX 6.1 (continued)
>
> - HCRA: Healthcare Resource Availability, component expressed as a percentile (1 = Best; 100 = Worst)
> - HIC: Health Insurance Coverage, component expressed as a percentile (1 = Best; 100 = Worst)
> - HCC: Healthcare Cost, component expressed as a percentile (1 = Best; 100 = worst)
>
> The intent in assessing these relationships is to test whether the relationship is as expected in terms of directionality (with increase in values of one variable what happens to values of the other variable), strength of relationship (indicated by absolute value of correlation coefficient), as well as whether this relationship is significant or not.
>
> In Exhibit 6.1, all possible relationships between pairs of variables have been generated. We focus on just the relationships of Years of Potential Life Lost under age 75 (YPPL_75) and the other variables which are seen in the first row of data. The first figure is the relationship of YPPL_75 with itself which is a perfect correlation of 1. Next, because YPPL_75 is a global measure of health and is related to both disability and economic distress, we see that there is moderately high correlation with both these variables. Because these variables have been modified to have higher values indicating worse states, the direction of correlation is positive, that is, as years of potential life lost increases, so does the worsening of these two variables of disability and economic distress. Also, this relationship is significant and does not occur by chance.
>
> There is moderate correlation (~0.5) between YPLL and the HCCA Index as well as between YPLL and the HCC component of this index, while there is weak correlation (~0.3) between YPLL and the HCRA component of the HCCA Index as well as between YPLL and the HIC component of this Index. As expected, with increasing YPLL, there is worsening of the HCCA Index as well as its components. The relationships between YPLL and the HCAA Index as well as its components are also significant and not a chance occurrence.

6.1 Exploring Relationships and Patterns

A good start to exploring relationships and patterns in data is described in Box. 6.1. Here, to ensure that the HCCA Index behaves in expected ways, the researchers use correlations to get a clearer idea of the relationship of this variable when seen together with another variable. Based on prior expectations, the researchers hypothesize relationships of this index with a global health outcome measure (years of potential life lost) to establish that indeed, as health outcome worsens, so does this index. The numerical value of this correlation coefficient also provides us with a magnitude of the strength of relationship, while the probability of this relationship not occurring by chance is confirmed through the level of significance.

In healthcare, decision-making is often based on exploring patterns and relationships. This exploration starts with the most basic depiction of data within a scatterplot and is then formalized using correlations and regression. When we are exploring and formalizing these relationships, it is worth clarifying at the start that "correlation" is not the same as "causation." Correlation helps us to confirm that a relationship between two variables is there and that this relationship has not occurred by chance. This is not the same as one variable causing changes in another variable. In order to establish causation, we need randomized studies that can confirm an intervention prior to the effect taking place.

A useful way to start to look at patterns in your dataset is through a scatterplot. In a scatterplot, we get a good visualization of the relationship between two variables in our dataset. This visualization then serves as a stepping stone to exploring further this relationship between the two variables and then applying certain metrics to this visualization and relationship to better interpret this relationship as well as use this information for predictions. In a nutshell, this is what correlation and regression are all about.

6.2 Scatterplot and Correlation

Exploring relationships begins with certain questions rather than just trying to put two variables together in the hope of then testing and finding a relationship—the classic kitchen sink analysis! In Dataset 3, our example, dataset based on Hospital Consumer Assessment of Healthcare Providers and Systems (HCAHPS) survey from Veterans Administration (VA) facilities, we have 11 variables. These are composite variables based on individual patient responses to surveys that covered several parts of the patient care experiences in these facilities. In order to explore the relationship among variables in this dataset, we consider possible relationships that "hang together" before we develop a scatterplot. In thinking through this relationship, it is a good idea to think of which variable affects the other, namely, which is the independent (x) and which is the dependent (y) variable.

Consider the variables "patients who understood their care" and "patients who rated the facility 9 or 10." Is there a possible relationship here? It is quite

Tutorial video for Section 6.2 is available by accessing the following url: https://connect .springerpub.com/content/book/978-0-8261-5028-8/chapter/ch11

possible that patients who understood their care will rate the facility higher. In this possible relationship, it is also likely that the independent variable here is "patients who understood their care" and the dependent variable is "patients who rated the facility 9 or 10." Given this theoretical possibility of relationship, let us visualize this relationship through a scatterplot.

In the worksheet containing the data, select the two columns containing data on "patients who understood their care" and "patients who rated the facility 9 or 10." After selecting all the data in these two columns—including the labels—click on "Insert" on the toolbar (Figure 6.1). In the ribbon under "Insert," find "Charts" and click on the "down arrow" next to Charts. In the window that opens, there are tabs for "Recommended Charts" and "All Charts"—click on "All Charts." Scroll down the list of charts till you find "X Y Scatter." Choose this as the chart type. You will notice that the first scatter-plots the values as two separate series for "Understood Care" and "Rating of 9 or 10" while the next scatter does not plot these values separately for the two series. Choose the second scatterplot.

Once you make your choice, the scatterplot may appear to disappear. Scroll through your worksheet and the scatterplot is likely to be at the top of the work-sheet. This scatterplot may at first appear tiny; go ahead and click on the scat-terplot and drag any of the outer corners to expand the size of this scatterplot.

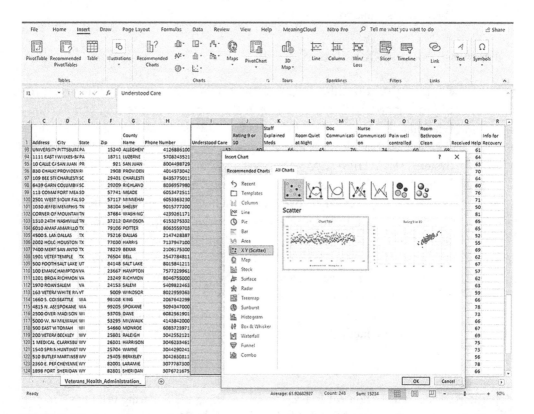

FIGURE 6.1 Inserting scatterplot.

Immediately discernible in this scatter is the upward or positive relationship between "Understood Care" and "Rating of 9 or 10." What this means is that as the values of "Understood Care" increase, so does the associated value of "Rating of 9 or 10." This is the theoretical relationship that we had started with and this visualization appears to bear out this relationship. Depending on the choice of variables, it is quite possible that other relationships may occur. A negative or inverse relationship indicates that as values of the independent variable increase, associated values of the dependent variable decrease. Or, there could be no relationship between our chosen independent and dependent variables.

6.2.1 Adding Trend Line to Scatterplot

We have a visual representation of the relationship between our chosen independent and dependent variables. However, we need some estimation of the measure of relationship. One way to do this estimation is through the trend line option in scatterplot (Figure 6.2). Go ahead and right click on any of the data points on the scatterplot. In the options that are displayed, choose "Add Trendline." Making this choice will open a panel "Format Trendline." In this panel, there are various options for our trend line to model the relationship. Based on what the relationship looks like on the scatterplot, we can see which option of trend line best fits with the scatterplot. Most of these options would require a more in-depth understanding of special relationships that are beyond the scope of this text. The linear option appears to fit our data well

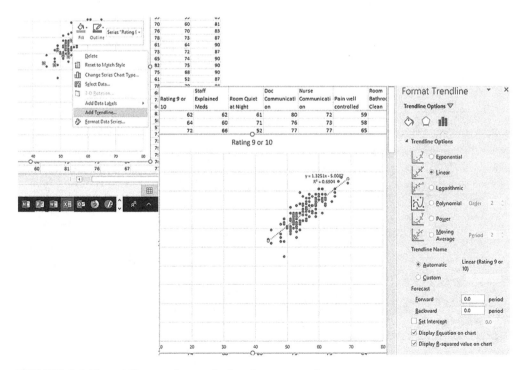

FIGURE 6.2 Trend line and correlation in scatterplot.

and it also lends itself to easier interpretation. Go ahead and choose the linear option and scroll down to the bottom of this panel and make sure to check the boxes for "Display Equation on Chart" and "Display R-Squared Value on Chart" and close this panel by clicking on the "X" at the top of this panel.

With these choices, now we see the trend line on our scatterplot as well as an equation and an R^2 value. We will come to the equation and interpret the R^2 value when we discuss regressions later in this chapter.

In order to get the coefficient of correlation or R or Multiple R, we need to click on "Data" on the toolbar and "Data Analysis" in the ribbon (Figure 6.3). In the Statistical Analysis and Tool panel that opens, scroll up and choose "Correlation." In the "Correlation" tab, the input range is the X (independent—understood care) and Y (dependent—rating of 9 or 10) variables together. Make this selection by choosing the "up arrow" next to "Input range," making sure to select the two columns, including the first row containing the data label. Click on the "down arrow" to make sure that your selected data range is in the "Input Range." Next, because our data are in columns, select "Column" for "Grouped by" and make sure to check the box against "Labels in First Row." The default option for this output is a new worksheet. If this is what you want, go ahead and click "OK."

The output of correlation is in a new worksheet. Go ahead and access this new worksheet (Figure 6.3). The correlation output shows a 2 by 2 table that has both variables displayed in the rows and columns. Because there is a perfect

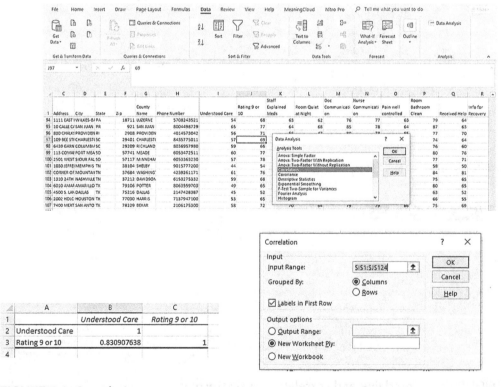

FIGURE 6.3 Correlation.

correlation between each variable in the row and column, the diagonal has the value 1. The correlation between "Understood Care" and "Rating of 9 or 10" is 0.8309. Because the correlation coefficient ranges from −1 to +1, this represents a highly positive relationship between these two variables. In characterizing this relationship, we need to account for not just the absolute value of this number but also the context and field (healthcare) to which it is being applied.

6.3 Regression

Moving on to regressions, think of regression as the development of a model that is attempting to explain the relationship between two or more variables. Formalized thus, it extends correlations and gives us greater confidence in interpreting results of this relationship analysis. It starts with a question such as: Is there a relationship between readmissions at a hospital and high postoperative utilization? This question is explored by Anderson, Golden, Jank, and Wasil (2012) in their study based on data from an academic medical center in the United States. Based on their study and using regression analysis, they were able to demonstrate that at 94% utilization rate, each additional bed increased probability of readmission by 0.35%. Similarly, we might have other questions that can be explored using regression analysis.

Let us now take up the regression equation and how to interpret and use the information from regression equations. We will start with a simple linear regression between one independent and one dependent variable and then consider multiple linear regression between several independent variables and one dependent variable (Kanji, 2009; Keller, 2006; Quirk, 2016). For more advanced topics in regression, please consult advanced statistical textbooks.

6.4 Single Linear Regression

In adding the trend line to our scatterplot (see Section 6.2.1, Adding Trend Line to Scatterplot) we got a sneak peek at a single linear regression equation: linear because this trend line option was chosen in fitting a trend line to our scatterplot, and single because it contained only one independent variable.

To access the regression option, we start with our data worksheet and click on "Data" on the toolbar and then on "Data Analysis" in the ribbon (Figure 6.4). This opens a panel with statistical tools and analysis. Scroll through this list till you see "Regression." Select "Regression" analysis. In the "Regression" tab, we can now go ahead and identify where our data are and

Tutorial video for Section 6.4 is available by accessing the following url: https://connect .springerpub.com/content/book/978-0-8261-5028-8/chapter/ch11

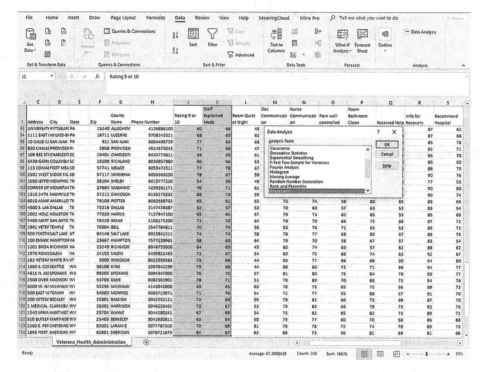

FIGURE 6.4 Regression.

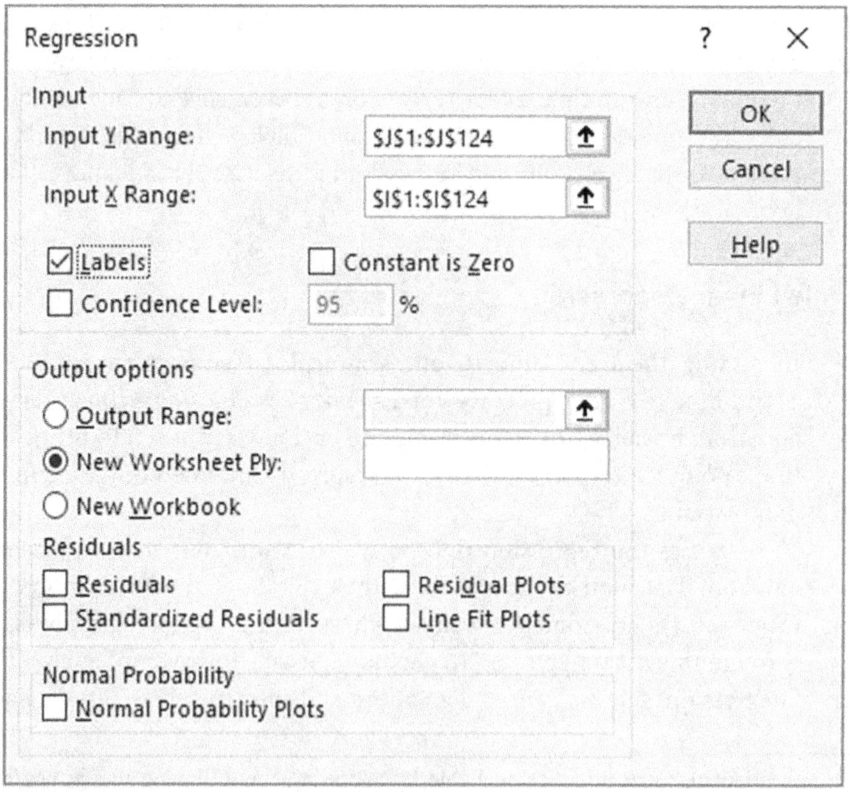

FIGURE 6.5 Choosing options for regression.

choose options for regression analysis (Figure 6.5). You will notice that we must input Y and X data ranges by choosing the relevant "up arrows." As discussed in the "Scatterplot and Correlation" section, the Y data range is the dependent variable (Rating of 9 or 10) and the X data range is the independent variable (Understood Care). Go ahead and make these selections for X and Y data ranges and make sure to include the column labels in the first row in your selection. Next, make sure to check the box next to "Labels." This alerts Excel to treat the first row of data as labels and not data. Notice that there is a box next to "Confidence Level." By default, this is set to 95%. In case this confidence level needs to be set to any other level (99%, 90%, etc.), only then should you check this box and make changes to this level. The default option is to have the output of this regression appear in a new worksheet. If this is what is desired, go ahead and click "OK" to run this regression.

Access the output of this regression by going to the new worksheet where this output has been sent. This regression output (Figure 6.6) contains several values and terms. We will focus on the key terms and values and their interpretation and application.

The first value is "Multiple R" or correlation coefficient. It has the same value (0.8309) as was obtained in the earlier section on correlation. As before, this is interpreted as a highly positive relationship between "understood care" and "rating of 9 or 10." Focus on the R^2 value for now. R^2 is the coefficient of determination. Its value gives a measure of the strength of relationship between the independent and dependent variables. Since its value is 0.6904, "understood care" (independent variable) explains 69.04% of the variation in "rating of 9 or 10" (dependent variable). This is a moderately high relationship between our independent and dependent variables.

In this first panel on "Regression Statistics," the adjusted R^2 is reported and discussed when we use multiple independent variables. Note that the "observations" alert us to the sample size—always a good idea to check that you have selected your entire sample.

SUMMARY OUTPUT

Regression Statistics	
Multiple R	0.830907638
R Square	0.690407503
Adjusted R Square	0.687848887
Standard Error	4.236336438
Observations	123

ANOVA

	df	SS	MS	F	Significance F
Regression	1	4842.630485	4842.63	269.8363	1.35316E-32
Residual	121	2171.532116	17.94655		
Total	122	7014.162602			

	Coefficients	Standard Error	t Stat	P-value	Lower 95%	Upper 95%	Lower 95.0%	Upper 95.0%
Intercept	-5.008728437	4.487036522	-1.11627	0.26652	-13.89200074	3.87454387	-13.8920007	3.87454387
Understood Care	1.325080475	0.08066628	16.4267	1.35E-32	1.165380296	1.484780654	1.165380296	1.484780654

FIGURE 6.6 Regression output.

Next, in the analysis of variance (ANOVA) panel, the "Significance F" value of 1.353.E-32 is a very small number—decimal place followed by 31 zeros. This is the probability of this F-Statistics. Because it is much smaller than 0.05 (or 5%), we reject the null hypothesis of no relationship between "Understood Care" (independent variable) and "Rating of 9 or 10" (dependent variable).

6.4.1 Predictions From Single Linear Regression

Moving down to the last panel of this output, we have the coefficients for "Intercept" and "Understood Care." These coefficients are used to form the regression equation:

Rating of 9 or 10 $= 1.325 \times$ Understood Care $- 5.009$

Because this is a linear regression equation, it is in the form of the equation for a line with the coefficient on "Understood Care" giving us the slope of the line and the constant giving us the y-intercept of this line. Notice that this equation is the same as the regression equation that was plotted on our trend line (Figure 6.2). Inserting values of the independent variable (Understood Care) in this equation will give us predicted values of the dependent variable (Rating of 9 or 10). For instance, for a value of 50 for "Understood Care," this equation will give us a predicted value of 61.24 for "Rating of 9 or 10" (see equation subsequently).

Rating of 9 or 10 $= 1.325 \times 50 - 5.009$

Rating of 9 or 10 $= 66.25 - 5.009$

Rating of 9 or 10 $= 61.24$

6.4.2 Testing Regression Coefficient

Finally, in this last panel of output, we also have a test of the coefficients and the probability that they are different from zero—meaning: do they have any effect on our regression? The coefficients that we need to check are the coefficients for our independent variable—"Understood Care." It is not interesting to check if the intercept is zero or not as it is meaningless in terms of the effect of variables in our regression. The coefficient on the independent variable is tested through the t-statistic and the corresponding probability (p value) and confidence interval (lower and upper bounds). In this regression, the coefficient for "Understood Care" is 1.325 with a probability of 1.35E-32—an infinitely small probability of a decimal point followed by 31 zeros. Because this probability is well below 5%, we fail to accept (reject) the null hypothesis that the coefficient on "Understood Care" is zero. This is also confirmed by making sure that zero is not in the 95% lower and upper bounds.

Based on this regression analysis, we conclude that our model explains almost 70% of the variation in our dependent variable "Rating of 9 or 10" and that there is a strong relationship between our independent variable ("Understood Care") and dependent variable. Also, "Understood Care" is a significant predictor in this model.

6.5 Multiple Regression

As the name suggests, "multiple regression" is regression that includes multiple (not single) independent variables to try to better explain the relationship in a regression model. Continuing with our example used for single linear regression, let us consider other available variables that could possibly explain the dependent variable—"Rating of 9 or 10." Among the remaining variables, it is plausible that "Room Quiet at Night," "Doctor Communication," and "Recommend Hospital" would be other independent variables that could be associated with the patient giving a "Rating of 9 or 10."

In order to use these variables for multiple regression, we need to ensure that the data columns are contiguous for the independent variables. Make sure to insert enough empty columns next to the single independent variable "Understood Care" and then cut and paste the other independent variables next to "Understood Care" and in columns adjacent to each other. This means that we have included "Understood Care," "Room Quiet at Night," "Doctor Communication," and "Recommend Hospital" in adjacent cells. Once the independent variables are in contiguous cells, we can go ahead check the correlation among these identified independent variables. Proceed as in Figure 6.3. The correlation output (Figure 6.7) shows us that the correlations among the independent variables range from 0.252 ("Room Quiet at Night" and "Doctor Communication") to 0.809 ("Understood Care" and "Recommend Hospital"). A few other correlations related to "Nurse Communication" are high (above 0.75). Because the correlations are not very high (>0.85), and if we are not going to use regression results for out-of-range (beyond the range of data for independent variables) predictions, we can proceed cautiously to the regression. Should the correlations be very high, one approach is to consider the correlations and try to figure out which variables are highly correlated, and thus not just creating redundancy in the model but also possibly other issues in the estimates and standard error. In this situation, suppose we consider for argument's sake that correlations that are greater than 0.75 are highly correlated. Then, in our correlation table (Figure 6.7), we notice that the variable "Recommend Hospital" is highly correlated with both "Understood Care" as well as "Nurse Communication" and that "Nurse Communication" and "Recommend Hospital" are highly correlated. We could then consider the relationships between these three variables and see which variables "hang together" better in this model. Based on this discussion, then consider

Tutorial video for Section 6.5 is available by accessing the following url: https://connect. springerpub.com/content/book/978-0-8261-5028-8/chapter/ch11

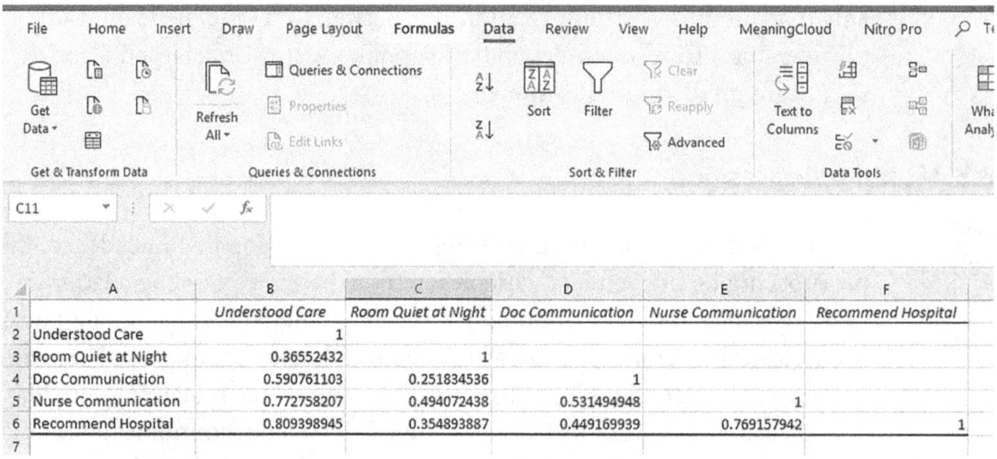

	Understood Care	Room Quiet at Night	Doc Communication	Nurse Communication	Recommend Hospital
Understood Care	1				
Room Quiet at Night	0.36552432	1			
Doc Communication	0.590761103	0.251834536	1		
Nurse Communication	0.772758207	0.494072438	0.531494948	1	
Recommend Hospital	0.809398945	0.354893887	0.449169939	0.769157942	1

FIGURE 6.7 Correlation of independent variables and multicollinearity.

dropping one of these three variables from our model. Note that dropping a variable should not be based solely on the correlations.

In making this choice of variables, we want to balance the association of these variables with the dependent variable ("Rating of 9 or 10") and ensure that the choice of independent variables is not highly correlated within the group of independent variables. This can lead to issues with multicollinearity that can affect the regression model and interpretation of results in this model. While this issue is beyond the scope of this text, there are resources such as from Penn State (Penn State Eberly College of Science, n.d.) that can provide pointers.

Now we can get started with running the regression model (Figures 6.4 and 6.5). Make sure that in selecting the "input X range" you select all the columns of data, including the first row with column labels. Once the multiple regression is run, we can access the output from the new worksheet (Figure 6.8).

The multiple regression output follows the pattern for single linear regression that we covered in the earlier section. The first value (0.9513) is "Multiple R" or correlation coefficient. As before, this is interpreted as a highly positive relationship between the dependent variable "Rating of 9 or 10" and our group of independent variables "Understood Care," "Room Quiet at Night," "Doctor Communication," "Nurse Communication," and "Recommend Hospital." Since we have more than one independent variable, we report the adjusted R^2 value because this adjusted value accounts for the use of multiple independent variables. Like R^2, the adjusted R^2 is the coefficient of determination. Its value gives a measure of the strength of relationship between the independent and dependent variables. Since its value is 0.9009, our group of independent variables explains 90.09% of the variation in "Rating of 9 or 10" (dependent variable). This is a strong relationship between our independent and dependent variables.

Note that the "observations" alert us to the sample size—always a good idea to check that you have selected your entire sample.

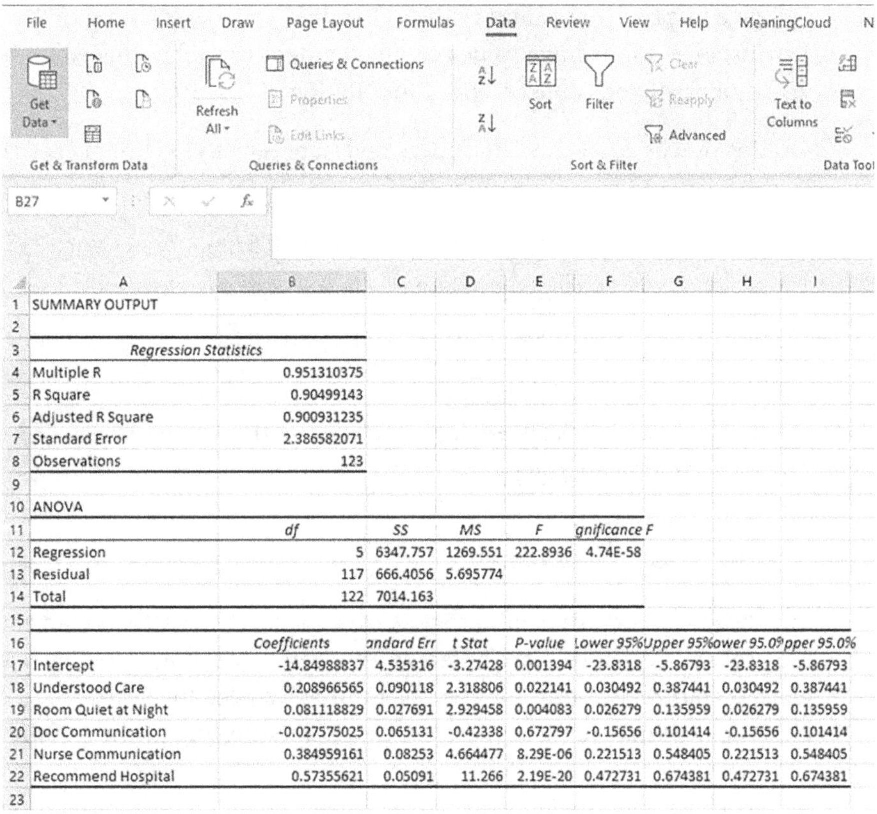

	A	B	C	D	E	F	G	H	I
1	SUMMARY OUTPUT								
2									
3	*Regression Statistics*								
4	Multiple R	0.951310375							
5	R Square	0.90499143							
6	Adjusted R Square	0.900931235							
7	Standard Error	2.386582071							
8	Observations	123							
9									
10	ANOVA								
11		*df*	*SS*	*MS*	*F*	*gnificance F*			
12	Regression	5	6347.757	1269.551	222.8936	4.74E-58			
13	Residual	117	666.4056	5.695774					
14	Total	122	7014.163						
15									
16		*Coefficients*	*andard Err*	*t Stat*	*P-value*	*Lower 95%*	*Upper 95%*	*ower 95.0%*	*pper 95.0%*
17	Intercept	-14.84988837	4.535316	-3.27428	0.001394	-23.8318	-5.86793	-23.8318	-5.86793
18	Understood Care	0.208966565	0.090118	2.318806	0.022141	0.030492	0.387441	0.030492	0.387441
19	Room Quiet at Night	0.081118829	0.027691	2.929458	0.004083	0.026279	0.135959	0.026279	0.135959
20	Doc Communication	-0.027575025	0.065131	-0.42338	0.672797	-0.15656	0.101414	-0.15656	0.101414
21	Nurse Communication	0.384959161	0.08253	4.664477	8.29E-06	0.221513	0.548405	0.221513	0.548405
22	Recommend Hospital	0.57355621	0.05091	11.266	2.19E-20	0.472731	0.674381	0.472731	0.674381
23									

FIGURE 6.8 Multiple regression output.

Next, in the ANOVA panel, the "Significance F" value of 4.74.E-58 is a very small number—decimal place followed by 57 zeros. This is the probability of this F-Statistics. Because it is much smaller than 0.05 (or 5%), we reject the null hypothesis of no relationship between our group of independent variables and "Rating of 9 or 10" (dependent variable).

6.5.1 Predictions From Multiple Regression

Moving down to the last panel of this output, we have the coefficients for "Intercept" and the independent variables. These coefficients are used to form the regression equation:

$$\begin{aligned}\text{Rating of 9 or 10} = 0.2090 * (\text{Understood Care}) + 0.0811 \times (\text{Room Clean}) - \\ 0.0276 \times (\text{Doc Communication}) + 0.3850 \times \\ (\text{Nurse Communication}) + 0.5736 \times \\ (\text{Recommend Hospital}) - 14.8499\end{aligned}$$

Inserting values of the independent variables, based on their ranges in our dataset (to offset any issues on account of multicollinearity) in this equation, will give us predicted values of the dependent variable ("Rating of 9 or 10"). For instance, for average values of independent variables, this equation will give us a predicted value of 59.424 for "Rating of 9 or 10."

$$\text{Rating of 9 or 10} = 0.2090 \times (\text{Understood Care}) + 0.0811 \times (\text{Room Clean}) -$$
$$0.0276 \times (\text{Doc Communication}) + 0.3850 \times$$
$$(\text{Nurse Communication}) + 0.5736 \times$$
$$(\text{Recommend Hospital}) - 14.8499$$
$$\text{Rating of 9 or 10} = 0.2090 \times (50) + 0.0811 \times (60) - 0.0276 \times (80) + 0.3850 \times$$
$$(70) + 0.5736 \times (60) - 14.8499$$
$$\text{Rating of 9 or 10} = 10.450 + 4.866 - 2.208 + 26.750 + 34.416 - 14.8499$$
$$\text{Rating of 9 or 10} = 59.424$$

6.5.2 Testing Regression Coefficients

Finally, in this last panel of output, we also have a test of the coefficients and the probability that they are different from zero—meaning: Do they have any effect on our regression? The coefficients that we need to check are the coefficients for our independent variables. It is not interesting to check if the intercept is zero or not, as it is meaningless in terms of the effect of variables in our regression. The coefficient on the independent variable is tested through the t-statistic and the corresponding probability (p value) and confidence interval (lower and upper bounds).

In this regression, the coefficient for "Understood Care" is 0.2090 with a probability of 0.022—a small probability. Because this probability is below 5%, we fail to accept (reject) the null hypothesis that the coefficient on "Understood Care" is zero. This is also confirmed by making sure that zero is not in the 95% lower and upper bounds.

Next, in this regression, the coefficient for "Room Clean" is 0.0811 with a probability of 0.004—a small probability. Since this probability is below 5%, we fail to accept (reject) the null hypothesis that the coefficient on "Room Clean" is zero. This is also confirmed by making sure that zero is not in the 95% lower and upper bounds.

The coefficient for "Doctor Communication" is −0.0276 with a probability of 0.673—a large probability. Because this probability is well above 5%, we fail to reject (accept) the null hypothesis that the coefficient on "Doctor Communication" is zero. This is also confirmed by making sure that zero is in the 95% lower and upper bounds.

In this regression, the coefficient for "Nurse Communication" is 0.3850 with a probability of 8029E-06—a small probability. Because this probability is well below 5%, we fail to accept (reject) the null hypothesis that the coefficient on "Nurse Communication" is zero. This is also confirmed by making sure that zero is not in the 95% lower and upper bounds.

Finally, in this regression, the coefficient for "Recommend Hospital" is 0.5736 with a probability of 2.19E-20—a very small probability. Since this probability is well below 5%, we fail to accept (reject) the null hypothesis that the coefficient on "Recommend Hospital" is zero. This is also confirmed by making sure that zero is not in the 95% lower and upper bounds.

Based on this regression, we can conclude that our regression model explains over 90% of the variation in our dependent variable "Rating of 9 or 10" and that there is a strong relationship between the combined independent variables and this dependent variable. Coming to the effects of individual independent variables, it is found that "Doctor Communication" is not a significant predictor in this model while "Recommend Hospital" and "Nurse Communication" are the most significant predictors.

6.6 Revisiting Missing Values

In Chapter 2, Working in Excel® and Importing Healthcare Data, we discussed the issue of missing data. The section, "Approaches to Missing Data" in this chapter pointed out some approaches to addressing this issue and that replacing missing values with averages is not advisable. Instead, the use of imputations for missing data is recommended. Here is where predictions from multiple regression (earlier in this chapter) can be used.

Let us start with some hypothetical VA facilities that are missing values on the variable "Rating of 9 or 10" (Figure 6.9). If we replace the missing value for these three facilities with the average value for "Rating of 9 or 10"—*not* a recommended approach—we would have replaced the three missing values with the average of 68.43.

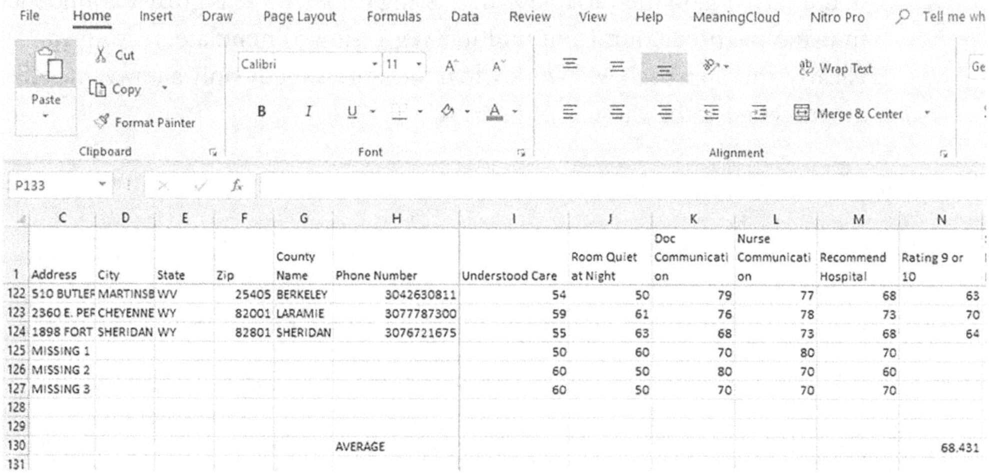

	C	D	E	F	G	H	I	J	K	L	M	N
1	Address	City	State	Zip	County Name	Phone Number	Understood Care	Room Quiet at Night	Doc Communication	Nurse Communication	Recommend Hospital	Rating 9 or 10
122	510 BUTLEF	MARTINSB	WV	25405	BERKELEY	3042630811	54	50	79	77	68	63
123	2360 E. PEF	CHEYENNE	WY	82001	LARAMIE	3077787300	59	61	76	78	73	70
124	1898 FORT	SHERIDAN	WY	82801	SHERIDAN	3076721675	55	63	68	73	68	64
125	MISSING 1						50	60	70	80	70	
126	MISSING 2						60	50	80	70	60	
127	MISSING 3						60	50	70	70	70	
128												
129												
130						AVERAGE						68.431
131												

FIGURE 6.9 Missing values and regression.

Tutorial video for Section 6.6 is available by accessing the following url: https://connect.springerpub.com/content/book/978-0-8261-5028-8/chapter/ch11

We do have an alternative. Our multiple regression model (Figure 6.8) with "Rating of 9 or 10" as the dependent variable, explained over 90% of the variation in "Rating of 9 or 10." We can use the regression equation for this model and use the values of the independent variables separately for each of our three hypothetical VA facilities missing values for "Rating of 9 or 10." In the regression equations that follow, we can replace the independent variables with their values to get the predicted value for the first VA facility with a missing value for "Rating of 9 or 10."

$$
\begin{aligned}
\text{Rating of 9 or 10} = {} & 0.2090\times(\text{Understood Care})+0.0811\times(\text{Room Clean}) \\
& -0.0276\times(\text{Doc Communication})+0.3850\times \\
& (\text{Nurse Communication})+0.5736\times \\
& (\text{Recommend Hospital})-14.8499
\end{aligned}
$$

$$
\begin{aligned}
\text{Rating of 9 or 10} = {} & 0.2090\times(50)+0.0811\times(60)-0.0276\times \\
& (70)+0.3850\times(80)+0.5736\times(70)-14.8499
\end{aligned}
$$

$$\text{Rating of 9 or 10} = 10.450 + 4.866 - 1.932 + 30.8 + 40.152 - 14.8499$$

$$\text{Rating of 9 or 10} = 69.487$$

These regression equations can be repeated separately for each of the other two VA facilities that are missing values for "Rating of 9 or 10." In this way, replacing the independent variables with the values of the independent variables for these facilities results in imputation of the missing values (Figure 6.10). Notice that replacing the missing values in this way, varies the values and is very different from just using the average value to replace these three missing values. Because this is based on a model that explains more than 90% of the variation in the variable with missing values, there is greater confidence in using the prediction from multiple regression to populate missing values. Clearly, this approach will work when there are already only a few values that are missing for the variable of interest.

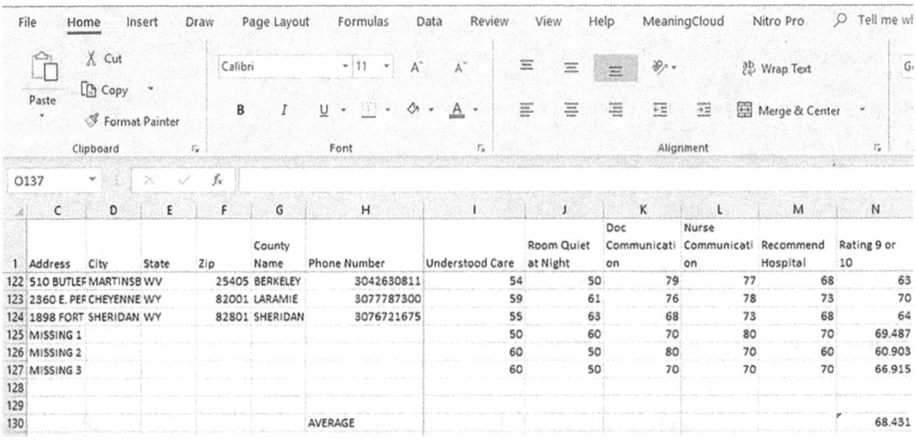

	C	D	E	F	G	H	I	J	K	L	M	N
1	Address	City	State	Zip	County Name	Phone Number	Understood Care	Room Quiet at Night	Doc Communication	Nurse Communication	Recommend Hospital	Rating 9 or 10
122	510 BUTLEF	MARTINSB	WV	25405	BERKELEY	3042630811	54	50	79	77	68	63
123	2360 E. PEF	CHEYENNE	WY	82001	LARAMIE	3077787300	59	61	76	78	73	70
124	1898 FORT	SHERIDAN	WY	82801	SHERIDAN	3076721675	55	63	68	73	68	64
125	MISSING 1						50	60	70	80	70	69.487
126	MISSING 2						60	50	80	70	60	60.903
127	MISSING 3						60	50	70	70	70	66.915
128												
129												
130						AVERAGE						68.431

FIGURE 6.10 Missing values imputed with predicted values.

6.7 Competency Development

The relationship of Years of Potential Life Lost below 75 years of age to dimensions of access to health professionals and facilities, health insurance coverage, and costs of healthcare are explored in Box. 6.1 through the HCCA Index in the Appalachian region. Here the Index itself is posited through frameworks such as social determinants of health to have a relationship with health outcomes. In order to establish this relationship, secondary data based on access to health professionals and facilities, health insurance coverage and costs of healthcare, and years of potential life lost below 75 years of age are tested. This testing is to establish three aspects of the relationship—directionality, strength, and statistical significance. Here, the use of a framework or model, to hypothesize the pattern of relationship between determinants of health and health outcomes, is a direct application of the competency domain of critical thinking.

A hypothesized relationship is not based on just hope and prayer; rather it is established through a framework or model. Next, we start the process of exploring this relationship by looking at basic patterns between variables through a scatterplot. At this stage, it is necessary to also distinguish between dependent and independent variables prior to invoking the scatterplot option in Excel charts. This visual representation is then concretized through inserting the trend line option in Excel to model the relationship between the variables through an equation as well as R^2 value. These steps provide application of competency domains of critical thinking as well as performance management.

Within Excel, in addition to the scatterplot, the Analysis ToolPak includes a routine that helps to undertake correlation between a dependent variable and an independent variable. Next, in order to better understand the relationship between a dependent variable and one or more independent variables, we use the option in Excel to run a regression to further test this relationship and assess all three aspects of the relationship—directionality, strength, and statistical significance. The resulting output from running a regression for a dependent variable and one or more independent variables can then be interpreted on all three aspects of the relationship in this model. In the example using the HCAHPS survey, the regression equation is also useful for making predictions of values of a dependent variable based on the regression model. Running and interpreting regression equations and its output and making predictions strengthen application of the competency domain of performance management.

When working with several independent variables in multiple regression, we need to be careful and test for multicollinearity between the independent variables and ensure that we do not complicate the regression and the validity of the test of relationships that it includes. This testing for multicollinearity enables application of skills related to the competency domain of problem-solving.

Regression models are also useful for addressing missing values in a dataset. This is achieved by running regression models and using predictions from the regression to replace missing values. This approach is more robust than either ignoring missing values or replacing missing values with average values. Using regression to address missing values furthers the application of skills from the competency domain of critical thinking and problem-solving.

In this chapter, through hypothesizing and exploring relationships, we focus on the critical thinking competency domain. Then, in running and interpreting correlations and regression, the focus is on the competency domains of critical thinking and performance management. Computing predictions, addressing multicollinearity, and imputing missing values bring the focus on competency domains of critical thinking and problem-solving.

6.8 Summary

Healthcare decision-making draws from hypothesized relationships between variables. The starting point for these relationships is based on theory as well as expectations on how different variables are likely to be related. In exploring these relationships, a scatterplot provides a visualization which can then be formed through computations of correlation and regression equations. The information that is contained in regression (single and multiple) outputs is applied to computing predictions as well as explaining the variation in dependent variable that is explained by the independent variables. Identifying and beginning to address multicollinearity helps to refine models of regression. Finally, multiple regression equations are used to provide predictions that can impute missing values when these are few and far between.

6.9 Discussion Questions

6.9.1 When trying to assess relationship between variables, how do you develop a hypothesized relationship?

6.9.2 If correlation is not causality, what is it? Explain.

6.9.3 Do regression models have any role to play in explaining variations in the dependent variable? Explain with an example.

6.9.4 In undertaking multiple regression models, an underlying concern is with multicollinearity. Use an example to explain what multicollinearity is.

6.9.5 What role do multiple regression models play in missing data? Explain.

⊙ 6.10 Practice Problems

All datasets required for the practice problems are available for download at http://connect.springerpub.com/content/book/978-0-8261-5028-8.

6.10.1 In Dataset 3, we are interested in understanding the outcome "Pain well controlled." To better understand this outcome, do the following:

a. Develop a scatterplot of this outcome with an independent variable from this dataset that you think explains "Pain well controlled." In this scatterplot, include a trend line with the regression equation. What do you conclude from this scatterplot?

b. Next, use the identified independent variable from "a" to run a single linear regression for "Pain well controlled." Interpret this regression and write the regression equation. Use this regression equation to predict the value of "Pain well controlled" for the average value of your independent variable.

c. Develop your regression model from "b" further by including two additional independent variables. Justify your choice of independent variables and check the correlation between these independent variables.

d. Use these three independent variables in a multiple regression for the outcome "Pain well controlled."

e. Interpret this regression and write the regression equation.

f. Use this regression equation to predict the value of "Pain well controlled" for the average values of your independent variables.

6.10.2 In Dataset 3, we are interested in understanding the variable "Recommend Hospital." To better understand this variable, do the following:

a. Develop a scatterplot of this outcome with an independent variable from this dataset that you think explains "Recommend Hospital." In this scatterplot, include a trend line with the regression equation. What do you conclude from this scatterplot?

b. Next, use the identified independent variable from "a" to run a single linear regression for "Recommend Hospital." Interpret this regression and write the regression equation. Use this regression equation to predict the value of "Recommend Hospital" for the average value of your independent variable.

c. Develop your regression model from "b" further by including two additional independent variables. Justify your choice of independent

---

⊙ Tutorial videos provided for Practice Problems 6.10.1—6.10.7 can be accessed by accessing the following url: https://connect.springerpub.com/content/book/978-0-8261-5028-8/chapter/ch11

variables and check the correlation between these independent variables.

d. Use these three independent variables in a multiple regression for the variable "Recommend Hospital."

e. Interpret this regression and write the regression equation.

Use this regression equation to predict the value of "Recommend Hospital" for the average values of your independent variables.

6.10.3 In Dataset 12, we are interested in understanding the outcome "% in Fair/Poor Health." To better understand this outcome—

a. Develop a scatterplot of this outcome with an independent variable from this dataset that you think explains "% in Fair/Poor Health." In this scatterplot, include a trend line with the regression equation. What do you conclude from this scatterplot?

b. Next, use the identified independent variable from "a" to run a single linear regression for "% in Fair/Poor Health." Interpret this regression and write the regression equation. Use this regression equation to predict the value of "% in Fair/Poor Health" for the average value of your independent variable.

c. Develop your regression model from "b" further by including two additional independent variables. Justify your choice of independent variables and check the correlation between these independent variables.

d. Use these three independent variables in a multiple regression for the outcome "% in Fair/Poor Health."

e. Interpret this regression and write the regression equation.

Use this regression equation to predict the value of "% in Fair/Poor Health" for the average values of your independent variables.

6.10.4 In Dataset 13, the variable "Communication With Nurses" is missing some values.

a. Undertake a multiple regression model with "Communication With Nurses" as your dependent variable and at least two or three independent variables.

b. Use the regression equation to get predicted values for the missing "Communication With Nurses" values.

6.10.5 In Dataset 13, the variable "Quietness of Hospital Environment" is missing some values.

a. Undertake a multiple regression model with "Quietness of Hospital Environment" as your dependent variable and at least two or three independent variables.

b. Use the regression equation to get predicted values for the missing "Quietness of Hospital Environment" values.

6.10.6 As a health policy lobbying group, you are interested in better understanding health insurance coverage as part of healthcare reform. Use Dataset 9 to better understand the variable "Percentage Point Decrease in Uninsured Rate 2010-15." To better understand this variable, do the following:

a. Develop a scatterplot of this outcome with an independent variable from this dataset that you think explains "Percentage Point Decrease in Uninsured Rate 2010-15." In this scatterplot, include a trend line with the regression equation. What do you conclude from this scatterplot?

b. Next, use the identified independent variable from "a" to run a single linear regression for "Percentage Point Decrease in Uninsured Rate 2010-15." Interpret this regression and write the regression equation. Use this regression equation to predict the value of "Percentage Point Decrease in Uninsured Rate 2010-15" for the average value of your independent variable.

c. Develop your regression model from "b" further by including two additional independent variables. Justify your choice of independent variables and check the correlation between these independent variables.

d. Use these three independent variables in a multiple regression for the outcome "Percentage Point Decrease in Uninsured Rate 2010-15."

e. Interpret this regression and write the regression equation.

f. Use this regression equation to predict the value of "Percentage Point Decrease in Uninsured Rate 2010-15" for the average values of your independent variables.

6.10.7 Given the ongoing policy discussion about the public and private financing of health insurance coverage, you have been tasked to better understand the health insurance market for individual health insurance plans. Use Dataset 9 to better understand the variable "Individual Market—Individuals With Marketplace Coverage (Q1 2016)." To better understand this variable, do the following:

a. Develop a scatterplot of this outcome with an independent variable from this dataset that you think explains "Individual Market—Individuals With Marketplace Coverage (Q1 2016)." In this scatterplot, include a trend line with the regression equation. What do you conclude from this scatterplot?

b. Next, use the identified independent variable from "a" to run a single linear regression for "Individual Market—Individuals With Marketplace Coverage (Q1 2016)." Interpret this regression and write the regression equation. Use this regression equation to predict the value of "Individual Market—Individuals With Marketplace Coverage (Q1 2016)" for the average value of your independent variable.

   c. Develop your regression model from "b" further by including two additional independent variables. Justify your choice of independent variables and check the correlation between these independent variables.

   d. Use these three independent variables in a multiple regression for the outcome "Individual Market—Individuals With Marketplace Coverage (Q1 2016)."

   e. Interpret this regression and write the regression equation.

   f. Use this regression equation to predict the value of "Individual Market—Individuals With Marketplace Coverage (Q1 2016)" for the average values of your independent variables.

See Chapter 11, Video Tutorials and Answers to Practice Problems Using Healthcare Datasets in Excel®, for video answers to the practice problems.

References

Anderson, D., Golden, B., Jank, W., & Wasil, E. (2012). The impact of hospital utilization on patient readmission rate. *Health Care Management Science, 15*, 29–36. doi:10.1007/s10729-011-9178-3

Kanji, G. K. (2009). *100 statistical tests* (3rd ed., reprinted). London, UK: Sage Publications.

Keller, D. K. (2006). *The tao of statistics: A path to understanding (with no math).* Thousand Oaks, CA: Sage Publications.

Lane, N. M., Lutz, A. Y., Baker, K., Konrad, T. R., Ricketts, T. R., Randolph, R., & Beadles, C. A. (2012). *Health care costs and access disparities in Appalachia* [Research report]. Retrieved from https://www.arc.gov/assets/research_reports/HealthCareCostsandAccessDisparitiesinAppalachia.pdf

Penn State Eberly College of Science. (n.d.). Lesson 12: Multicollinearity & other regression pitfalls. Retrieved from https://onlinecourses.science.psu.edu/stat501/lesson/12

Quirk, T. J. (2016). *Excel 2016 for health services management statistics: A guide to solving practical problems.* New York: Springer.

VISUALIZATION AND SPATIAL ANALYSIS OF HEALTHCARE DATA USING 3D MAPS IN EXCEL®

LEARNING OBJECTIVES

- Identify purpose to drive visualization of data through maps
- Connect data display using maps to healthcare decision-making
- Use mapping capabilities within Excel
- Convert data to tables in preparation for display as maps
- Understand when to use specific data display within maps
- Customize maps and their display elements
- Develop scenes in maps to tell your data story
- Create tours to animate time series data
- Produce your scenes for print or video

In this chapter, we use 3D Maps in Excel to visualize and analyze data in three dimensions. In addition to three-dimensional maps, this feature within Excel uses time variable in data to visualize a video of data aggregation. The focus in this chapter is on the competency domains of critical thinking, information management, problem-solving, and communication.

7.1 Why and When to Map Data

Representing data on maps needs to be dictated by a purpose and the story that you want to convey. As Box 7.1 suggests, we have different options for

---

Throughout the chapter supplemental content is available for the datasets and tutorial videos. Video availability is denoted with an icon. To gain access to these items, please visit the following urls:

Datasets: https://connect.springerpub.com/content/book/978-0-8261-5028-8

⊙ Tutorial Videos: https://connect.springerpub.com/content/book/978-0-8261-5028-8/chapter/ch11

BOX 7.1 LOCATING DATA ON MAP

From times immemorial, humans have been fascinated with maps: maps that in ancient times showed trade routes to riches and goods from distant lands, to more modern times where we rely on maps (paper and digital) to guide us to places near and far. This fascination is driven by a deep-seated desire to find precise locations for places.

There are different ways to visualize data. Specialized software such as Tableau has taken the lead in making visualizations very pleasing and easy to use. In their *Visual Analysis Best Practices: A Guidebook*, they succinctly state: "when you want to show a location, use a map" (Tableau, n.d., p. 13). But just because we have geographical data does not mean we should put it on a map. "Here's why: maps, like all methods of visualization, are designed for a purpose. They tell *particular types of stories* well—but not all of them" (Bradshaw, n.d.).

Take for example Figures 7.1 and 7.2 here. Both these visualizations provide a very attractive display of the underlying data. The data in these two visualizations are arrayed neatly as horizontal bars in Figure 7.1 and as state boundaries in Figure 7.2. Which one is a better visualization? Yes, the bars will appeal to particular audiences and the maps to possibly others with some overlap between these two sets of audiences. What may

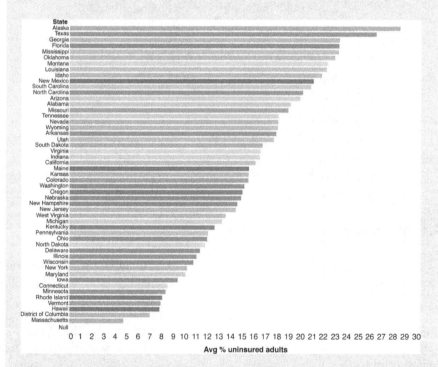

FIGURE 7.1 Average percentage of uninsured adults in the United States (2016).

(continued)

BOX 7.1 (*continued*)

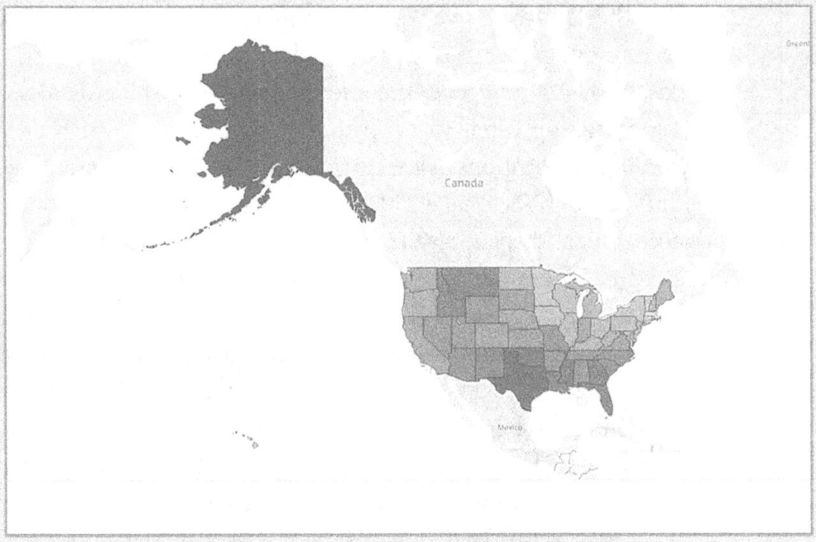

FIGURE 7.2 Geographical distribution of average percentage of uninsured adults in the United States (2016).

not be readily apparent is that the underlying data in both these figures are *exactly* the same. Data from County Health Rankings (County Health Rankings and Roadmaps, n.d.) are used in Tableau to generate these two figures. And to choose between the two visualizations is not a fair choice. Each of these figures serves a specific purpose and is created to that end. Figure 7.1 is ideal where we want to showcase the highs and lows of this data on average percentage of uninsured adults. The states with the highest uninsured rates—Alaska, Texas, Georgia, Florida, and Mississippi—are at the top and the states/districts with the lowest rates are at the bottom—Rhode Island, Vermont, Hawaii, District of Columbia, and Massachusetts. In Figure 7.2, the emphasis is on the geographical distribution of the states by average uninsured rates among adults. In this map, the gradation of gray tinting provides the range of uninsured rates with the darker gray indicating higher uninsured rates. Here the geographical distribution and clustering of high and low rates are readily apparent.

Thus, depending on what our purpose is and what story we want to communicate with our figures, we would choose between figures such as a horizontal bar graph or a map.

displaying data. The same underlying data on average uninsured adults in the United States lends itself to visualizing as a horizontal bar graph (Figure 7.1) or as a map (Figure 7.2). As with any visualization, the figure does not drive the visualization. Rather, it is the purpose and the story that we wish to convey through the underlying data.

A variety of specialized software such as Tableau has made the process of visualizing data very easy. However, rather than purchasing and learning another software, we will use some of the inbuilt capabilities in Excel to deliver on our purpose of depicting data through maps.

Based on our purpose, the use of maps to display data and analysis aids decision-making when we wish to focus on decisions such as identifying and addressing the locations of low uninsured rates (Figure 7.2) and possibly addressing this through regional efforts at coordinating health insurance markets. Such a geographical display of analyzed data would also aid in understanding and responding to market segmentation of healthcare services and identifying the distribution and spread of coverage as well as health outcome data.

Visual representation of data was covered using charts (Chapter 3, Identifying, Categorizing, and Presenting Healthcare Data Using Excel®). We did not cover maps within chart types as there is a powerful feature called 3D Maps embedded within Excel. To use 3D Maps or "Power Maps," as it was earlier referred to, you need data that include any location variable such as an address, city, state, country, and so on. Together with your data, 3D Maps use this location information to then transform your data in three dimensions using maps powered by Bing. This static feature within 3D Maps takes a dynamic turn when any time variable within your data is then used to develop a video tour of your data and how it changes over time. Let us explore these features within 3D Maps.

7.2 Converting Data to Tables

To get started, we will use the Hospital Consumer Assessment of Healthcare Providers and Systems (HCAHPS) survey from Veterans Administration (VA) facilities as our example. Go ahead and open Dataset 3. As we open this data in Excel, we notice that our dataset has several location variables—address, city, state, zip, and county name—in addition to data on composite measures on patient experiences. In order to get started with using 3D Maps, our data must be in the form of tables (Microsoft Office Support, n.d.). To do this, we go ahead and select the entire data, including the column headers. An easy way to do this selection is to place your cursor in the first cell (A1) and hold down the "Control" and "Shift" keys (together) and press the "right arrow" key. Next, while still holding down Control and Shift keys (together), press the "down arrow" key. Once the entire data are selected, go to the "Insert" menu in the toolbar and click on "Table" in the Tables group of the ribbon (Figure 7.3). In the "Create Table" menu that appears, make sure that the range includes your entire data and that there is a check next to "My table has headers." As soon as you click "OK," your data are transformed into a table (Figure 7.4) with each column header now displaying a "down arrow" next to the column.

Tutorial video for Sections 7.2 to 7.4 is available by accessing the following url: https://connect.springerpub.com/content/book/978-0-8261-5028-8/chapter/ch11

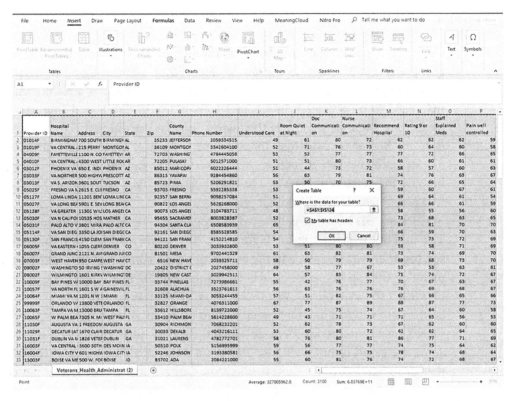

FIGURE 7.3 Converting data into tables.

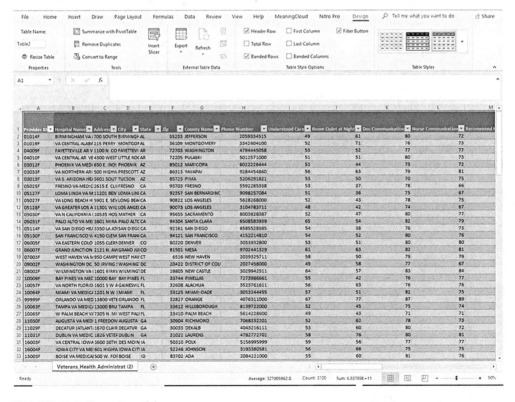

FIGURE 7.4 Data in tables.

7.3 Turn to 3D Maps

Go back to "Insert" on the toolbar and now on the ribbon look for the "Tours" group and find 3D Maps in this group (Figure 7.5). Depending on your version of Excel, 3D Maps, earlier referred to as "Power Maps," is a feature that may need to be activated. In Chapter 2, Working in Excel® and Importing Healthcare Data, we went over the instructions for activating this in the section on "Managing Add-Ins." In case your version of Excel does not show 3D Maps, follow the instructions for activating this Add-in. In this example, because the version of 3D Maps has been activated, you will notice that the "3D Maps" icon is active and not grayed.

Click on "3D Maps" to get started. As you invoke 3D Maps, you should see a picture of the globe appear (Figure 7.6). This is the 3D Map view and you see, together with the globe in the center, there is a contextual (for 3D Maps) menu on the top to use for a variety of options in 3D Maps. Next, the panel on the left shows "Tour 1" with "Scene 1" with a duration of 10 seconds. This is where we will add different visualizations and analysis and capture them as scenes, set a duration for them, and turn them into videos. In the center, just above the globe, is the "Field List" that has a listing of all the variables (fields) that are in our data table. These fields can be dragged and dropped in the panel to the right to be used for visualizations as well as categories and filters. In case we have a time field, this can be dragged to the field under "Time." Through this panel, we can use the icons under "Data" to change the visualization from the default of stacked columns to clustered columns, bubbles, or a heat map.

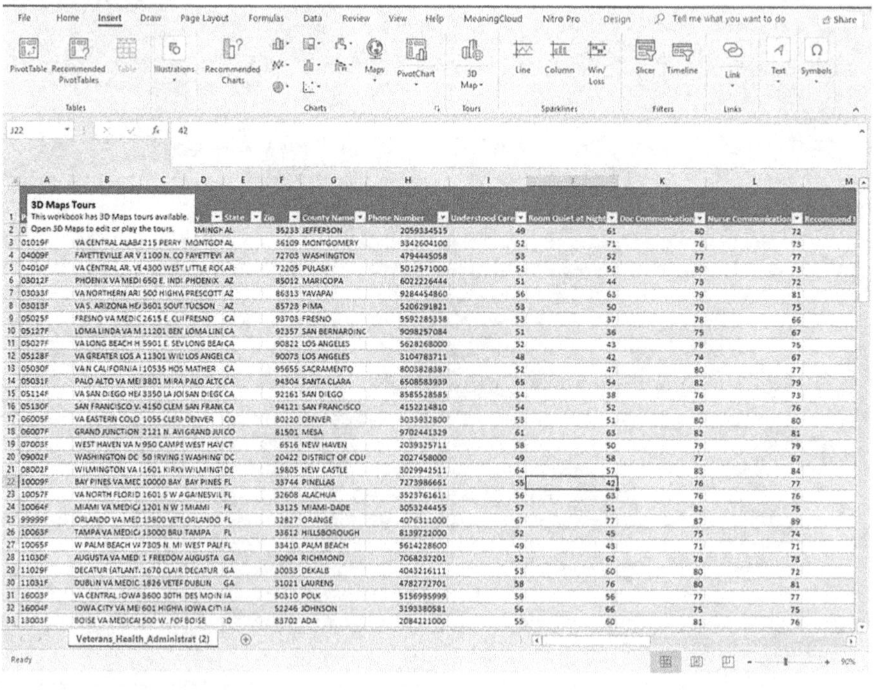

FIGURE 7.5 Start 3D maps.

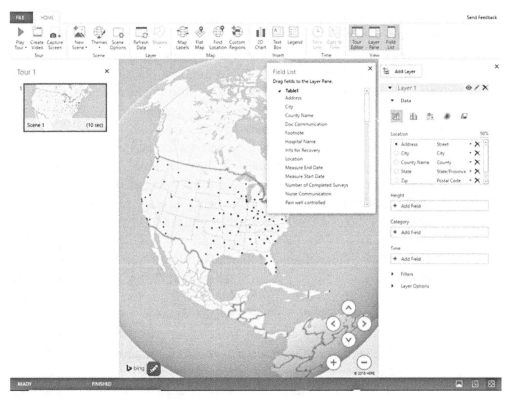

FIGURE 7.6 3D maps in Excel.

SOURCE: Map materials © 2019 HERE.

On our map, depending on the purpose of the visualization, we could choose the columns, bubbles, or heat map to display data. The choice of which of these three data displays to choose depends on the purpose and story we want to convey. For instance, the columns are a great way to display averages or achievement on a variable, while bubbles would be a good way to draw comparisons between different locations on the map. If we want to focus on density of data, then a heat map would show the intensity very well.

7.4 Steps in Visualizing 3D Maps

Now that our data are in 3D Maps, we can get started with the visualization. The first step is to check the mapping of location fields. Make sure that the mapping maintains correspondence between the fields in the dataset and the fields for locations that are in 3D Maps. In our dataset, we have address, city, county name, state, and zip. These are mapped on to street, city, county, state/province, and postal code. This mapping is accurate. In case the mapping was not accurate, go ahead and click the "down arrow" next to the field mapping and correct it. Any of the location fields can be used to represent information on the globe. Currently, it is displaying locations by "Address." Let us change this to "State."

Next, go to "Height." This represents the height of the bars that are used for representation of data fields. Click on "Add field" and choose "Number of completed surveys." By default, the sum of completed surveys by "State"—our chosen location level—is displayed. To the right of "Number of completed surveys" is a "down arrow." Clicking on it allows you to make changes to the aggregation. We can choose "average" such that we now have the average by state of HCAHPS surveys completed by patients.

We currently do not have categories in this dataset. However, if we were to create star ratings for any of the fields, these could potentially serve as categories by which to display data. However, for our dataset, we can add the field "State" as a filter. Using "State" as a filter will allow us to restrict the data to the chosen states. For now, we will keep all the states in our visualization.

At the bottom of our panel on the right is "Layer Options" (Figure 7.7). This is our gateway to modify the current chart elements that are displayed. Through "Layer Options" we can go ahead and change features such as the height, thickness, and color of the elements of our visualization. Go ahead and make changes and the bars immediately show the effect of these changes.

On the globe, at the lower right, you will see a set of four arrows and "+" and "−." The latter are used to zoom in and zoom out, respectively, while the arrows help to pan the globe on a variety of axes.

Our current visualization of the average number of completed surveys is the first scene in our tour. You will see this scene on the left panel with a

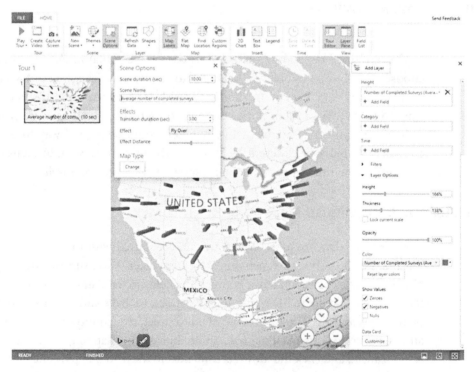

FIGURE 7.7 Adding scenes.

SOURCE: Map materials © 2019 HERE.

duration in seconds for which it is by default to play. If you hover over the time, it will display both a "play" button and a "cogwheel." Clicking on the play button will make the globe full screen and it will play the visualization. Clicking the cogwheel, or clicking on "Scene Options" in the ribbon, will bring up a panel that you can use to format some options. For this scene, we can go ahead and include a name for the scene and choose and select an effect "Fly Over." With these changes made, if you now click on the "play" button in the scene, or through the "Play Tour" option in the ribbon, you will get a sense of flying over this visualization as the video plays out.

If for some reason, for your purposes, you are more comfortable with two dimensions and not a three-dimensional globe, go ahead and chose "Flat Map" from the ribbon (Figure 7.8).

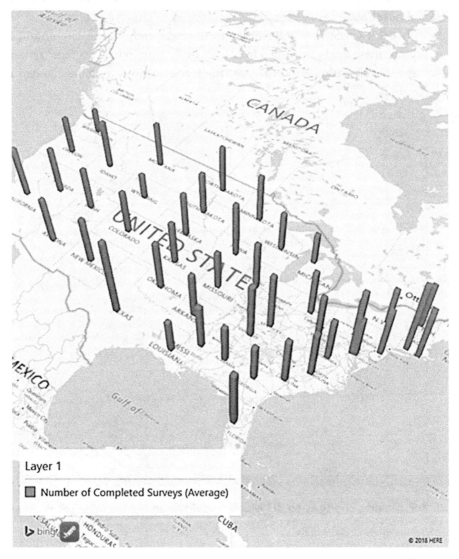

FIGURE 7.8 Flat maps.

SOURCE: Map materials © 2019 HERE.

7.5 Working With Scenes

Think of the scenes like a storyboard that you are going to use to tell a story. Each scene helps to move your story forward. We have set the stage by identifying the average number of completed surveys. This serves as the basis for identifying and highlighting key aspects of our data. For instance, based on the multiple regression model (Chapter 6, Checking Patterns in Healthcare Data Using Scatterplots, Correlations, and Regressions in Excel®) we found that the field "Recommend Hospital" and "Nurse Communication" were very significant predictors of "Rating of 9 or 10." We can add two scenes to display this information.

To add a scene, go ahead and click on "Add Scene" in the ribbon and then choose "World Map" (Figure 7.9). After this, go through the "Steps in Visualizing 3D Maps" (section mentioned previously). First, make sure to choose "State" as the location. Next, choose "clustered columns" as we will choose two fields—"Recommend Hospital" and "Nurse Communication." Once these fields are added to height, make sure to use "average" rather than the default "sum." After this, use the layout options to make changes to the

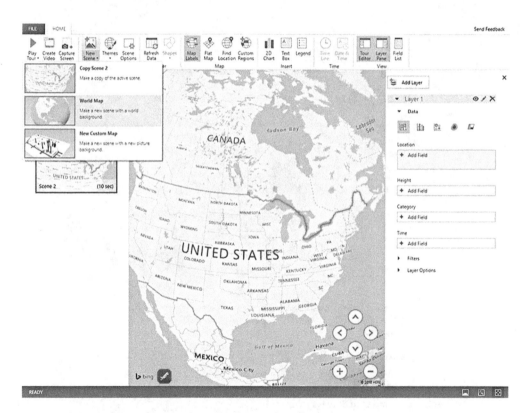

FIGURE 7.9 Making changes to 3D Maps visualization.

SOURCE: Map materials © 2019 HERE.

Tutorial video for Section 7.5 is available by accessing the following url: https://connect .springerpub.com/content/book/978-0-8261-5028-8/chapter/ch11

height, thickness, and color of the columns and click "Scene Options" to change the effect to circle.

Go ahead and add another scene to 3D Maps and for this scene use "State" as the location and choose "Rating of 9 or 10." Here, we will use the heat map for our data and make changes to format this scene as desired.

Once we are ready with all three scenes, go ahead and include legends from the ribbon in each of the scenes. Make sure to resize and position the legend such that it does not overlap your map. After this, use the "Play Tour" button on the ribbon to see how your scenes are playing out.

7.5.1 Duplicating Scenes and Using Filters

To see how filters work, go to scene 2 (Nurse Communication and Recommend Hospital) and click on "Add Scene." Now, instead of creating a new scene based on the world map, we will go ahead and duplicate scene 2 and use a filter here. Choose the option "Copy Nurse Communication and Recommend Hospital" and scene 2 is duplicated. If we want to reorder the scenes, simply drag and move scenes up or down to the desired location.

Coming to the duplicated scene—scene 3 currently. We go to the right panel beyond the globe and "Add Filter" and choose "State" in the field list. Seeing that our map visualization is very dense in the Northeast, we can choose to filter states in the Northeast and exclude other states from our visualization (Figure 7.10).

7.6 Including Time Element

Our current dataset has a field for time—"Measure Start Date" and "Measure End Date." However, both fields do not show any variability. In order to appreciate how a variable time field can be used dynamically within 3D Maps, for this example, we can go ahead and alter the "Measure Start Date." Note, this is *not* recommended for any data with which you are working and is being done only to show how a variable time field is used within 3D Maps.

Because we are altering data, to get started, we go ahead and create a copy of the existing worksheet so that we do not lose the original data. Once the copy is created, we rename this new worksheet "VHA Date Modified." In this worksheet, we will first select the entire data in the column "Measure Start Date" and right click and choose "Format Cell" and make sure that the data in this column are in a date format (Figure 7.11). For 3D Maps to recognize this field as a date field, the data must be formatted as "date." Once this is done, go ahead and change the dates in this column. In our example, the dates were changed for the last day of the month for 2017 for the first 12 entries—noting that not all months have 30 or 31 days and there is the special case for February! The

---

Tutorial video for Sections 7.5.1 to 7.6 is available by accessing the following url: https://connect.springerpub.com/content/book/978-0-8261-5028-8/chapter/ch11

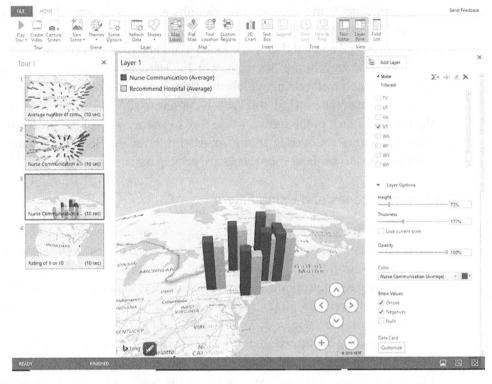

FIGURE 7.10 Using filters.

SOURCE: Map materials © 2019 HERE.

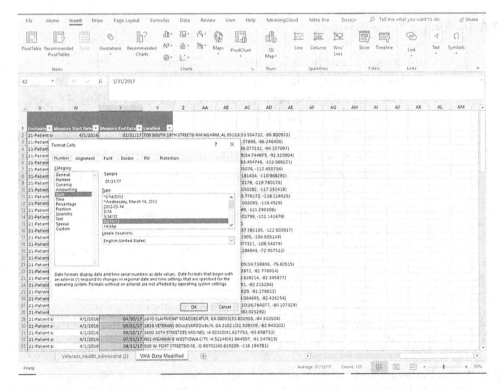

FIGURE 7.11 Formatting as date.

easiest way to then make changes in the remaining data is to copy this block of 12 cells and go ahead and paste it down the column in blocks of 12 cells.

Because our data are already available as a data table, as before (see section "Turn to 3D Maps") we choose "3D Maps" from the "Tour Group" under "Insert in the toolbar." Our earlier tour where we created a 3D Map is already here—since we are using the same data table. Go ahead and choose "New Tour." We follow through with the steps to add fields to the location such that they are mapped on to the location fields in 3D Maps (Figure 7.12). For "height," we will again choose "Number of Completed Surveys" and now we will keep the aggregation as "Sum." Finally, under "Time," go ahead and choose "Measure End Date." Notice that next to this field, there is a down arrow. Go ahead and click it. The time options that are revealed are to make a choice as to what time period we will be using for aggregating the data in this case on "Number of Completed Surveys." Because our date field is in months, we can choose either "month" or "quarter" for aggregation. Let us choose "month."

Notice that in the center of our screen, our globe now has a "play" button. This feature automatically appears anytime we include the time filed in 3D Maps. Go ahead and change any layout options such as height, thickness, and color. Once you are ready, go ahead and click on the "gear" button on the globe and make sure that the entire time period is available. Now go ahead and click on the "play" button and see the animation by month of the number of collected surveys.

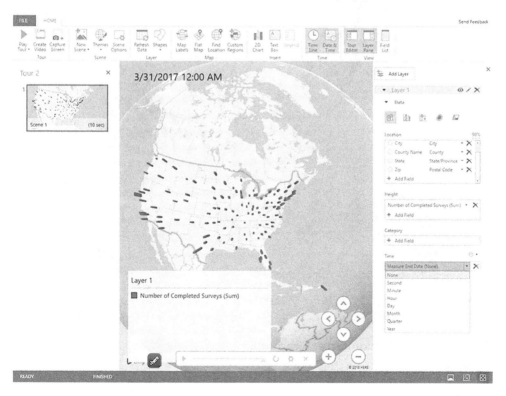

FIGURE 7.12 3D Maps using time data.

SOURCE: Map materials © 2019 HERE.

7.7 Production of Tour

If you are satisfied with the effect and the story that it is conveying, we can move into production. As part of the production process, you can modify the look and feel of the maps by choosing "Themes" from the ribbon. After this, the production of the story through the scenes can be done in two formats.

7.7.1 Print/Slide Production

Go ahead and pull in each scene one at a time and use the pan and zoom features to display the map as you would like. Once you are happy with the visualization, use the "Screen Capture" icon from the ribbon (Figure 7.13). This

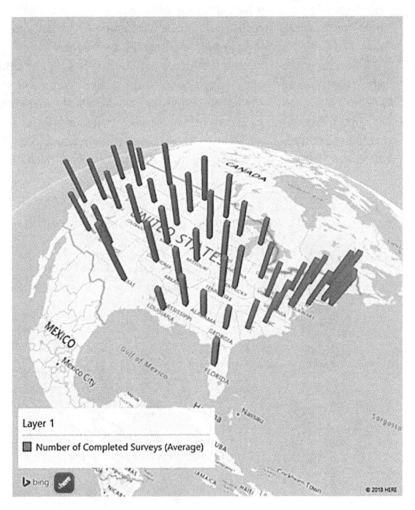

FIGURE 7.13 Production: Screen capture.

SOURCE: Map materials © 2019 HERE.

Tutorial video for Section 7.7 is available by accessing the following url: https://connect
.springerpub.com/content/book/978-0-8261-5028-8/chapter/ch11

"Screen Capture" copies your map to clipboard and you can paste this map in your slide or in a document. Repeat this for all scenes that you wish to capture.

7.7.2 Video Production

For producing your video, a variety of options for quality of video are available as well as adding a soundtrack to your production (Figure 7.14). These include producing a high-quality video as well as customizing it to a variety of platforms such as laptops and smartphones.

Once you are done with 3D Maps, go to "File" on the toolbar and click "Close." You can always come back to your 3D Map and the tour that you just created through your data table. Once you are in the data table, go ahead and choose "Insert" and click on "3D Maps." This will open 3D Maps and show you tours already created. If you want to continue working on your tour, click on the existing tour (Tour 1) and go ahead and make changes. Otherwise, simply create a new tour.

7.8 Competency Development

Box 7.1 highlights the conundrum in dealing with data that have a geographical basis. The ready instinct is to use maps to display these data. However, rather than being driven by instinct, it is best to take a step back and ponder

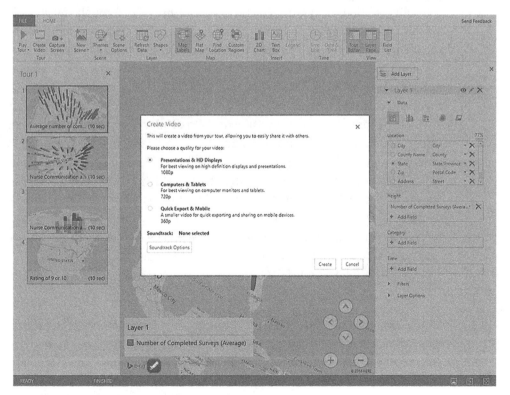

FIGURE 7.14 Production: Create video.

SOURCE: Map materials © 2019 HERE.

the question that you hope to answer with these data and then consider what is the best way to visualize the data—through a map or another table, figure, or chart. Thinking through the visualization and making sure that your visualization answers the question that you set out with help in applying skills form the competency domains of critical thinking and problem-solving.

Having settled on a question that can be visualized using maps, we need to ensure that our data also include one or more location variables such as city, county, state, country, and so on. If both these conditions are met, we can proceed to use the 3D Maps feature in Excel to visualize our data through static or dynamic maps. The starting point for using this 3D Maps feature in Excel is to first convert our data into tables. Depending on the purpose of the visualization, we could choose the columns, bubbles, or heat map to display data. Next, based on the question that we have set out to answer, we need to evaluate which of the three available data displays to choose. For instance, the columns are a great way to display averages or achievement on a variable, while bubbles would be a good way to draw comparisons between different locations on the map. If we want to focus on density of data, then a heat map would show the intensity very well. These steps in accessing and using the 3D Maps within Excel as well as choosing a specific data display provide application of skills from the competency domains of information management and problem-solving.

Having settled on the data display, we can proceed through the steps in visualizing the maps and create scenes and modify these scenes through targeted and purpose-driven use of filters as well as use time series data to develop videos of the data aggregating on our maps. These steps then provide application of skills from the competency domains of information management and communication.

Being purpose driven in choosing maps to display analyzed data and using this to aid healthcare decision-making, we are developing the competency domains of critical thinking and problem-solving. Next, in applying mapping capabilities in Excel and knowing when to use which features of map display, we are focusing on the competency domains of information management and problem-solving. The creation of scenes and tours as well as production of scenes for print and video develop the competency domains of information management and communication.

7.9 Summary

The decision to visualize data through maps in Excel is informed by the purpose behind the analysis of data such that it aids decision-making and does not distract from it. Excel has inbuilt capabilities in depicting geographical data through a variety of maps and elements. In order to use these capabilities, we start by converting the data into tables and then choosing specific ways—columns, bubbles, and heat maps—to display data using maps. Next, the focus on the purpose of data analysis and display helps to

*develop scenes to tell the story as well as create tours to animate time series data. Finally,
the production of scenes for print as well as video helps to communicate our data story.*

7.10 Discussion Questions

7.10.1 How would you choose to display your data through a graph or a map?

7.10.2 What kinds of healthcare decision-making lend themselves to using maps to display data?

7.10.3 Do you find it useful to visualize maps through videos or would you rather just see them as printed or digital maps? Why?

7.11 Practice Problems

All datasets required for the practice problems are available for download at http://connect.springerpub.com/content/book/978-0-8261-5028-8.

7.11.1 In Dataset 3, we are interested in understanding the geographical distribution of the issues highlighted by patients at a VA facility. Use the fields "Pain well controlled" and "Staff explained meds" to explore the geographical distribution.

a. Develop maps at the state level for these two issues.

b. Create categories for "highly recommend hospital" or "not highly recommend hospital" by using the 75th percentile as cutoff. Use "recommend high/not high" as a filter for your visualization.

c. Create scenes based on your visualization.

d. Based on your scenes, go ahead and use these scenes as images to explain the issues involved.

e. Use these scenes to develop a short video using these two fields.

f. What conclusions do you arrive at?

7.11.2 In Dataset 12, we are interested in understanding the geographical distribution of the issues highlighted by county. Use the fields "% physically inactive" and "% with access to exercise" to explore the geographical distribution.

a. Develop maps at the state level for these two issues.

b. Create categories for poor health or fair health by using the 75th percentile as cutoff for the variable "% in Fair/Poor Health." Use "fair/poor" as a filter for your visualization.

Tutorial videos provided for Practice Problems 7.11.1—7.11.6 can be accessed by accessing the following url: https://connect.springerpub.com/content/book/978-0-8261-5028-8/chapter/ch11

    c. Create scenes based on your visualization.

    d. Based on your scenes, go ahead and use these scenes as images to explain the issues involved.

    e. Use these scenes to develop a short video using these two fields.

    f. What conclusions do you arrive at?

7.11.3 In Dataset 12, we are interested in understanding the geographical distribution of the issues highlighted by county. Use the fields "physically unhealthy days" and "mentally unhealthy days" to explore the geographical distribution.

    a. Develop maps at the state level for these two issues.

    b. Create categories for poor health or fair health by using the 75th percentile as cutoff for the variable "% in Fair/Poor Health." Use "fair/poor" as a filter for your visualization.

    c. Create scenes based on your visualization.

    d. Based on your scenes, go ahead and use these scenes as images to explain the issues involved.

    e. Use these scenes to develop a short video using these two fields.

    f. What conclusions do you arrive at?

7.11.4 Use Dataset 11. From this file, use the data on crude rate to show how the states have changes over time. In your visualization use "male/female" as a filter. What does your visualization show?

7.11.5 As a journalist working on a story about the Affordable Care Act and its impact on health insurance rates at the state level, you are thinking about how best to include data on this topic for your write-up. You have access to Dataset 9. In this dataset, you are interested in understanding the geographical distribution of the fields "uninsured rate 2010%" and "uninsured rate 2015%" to explore their geographical distribution.

    a. Develop maps at the state level for these two issues.

    b. Use "State Expanded Medicaid 2016" as a filter for your visualization of "uninsured rate 2015%."

    c. Create scenes based on your visualization.

    d. Based on your scenes, go ahead and use these scenes as images to explain the issues involved.

    e. Use these scenes to develop a short video using these two fields.

    f. What conclusions do you arrive at?

7.11.6 You are working with a health policy advocacy group that wants to focus attention on the benefits of insurance coverage and how these have changed under the Affordable Care Act (ACA). As an analyst, you are thinking about how best to include data on this topic for your presentation. You have access to Dataset 9. In this dataset, you are interested in understanding the geographical distribution of the fields related to lifetime limits on health benefits pre-ACA and private coverage with no cost sharing for preventive services. Focus on a specific target population (total, children, adult males, or adult females) to explore their geographical distribution.

a. Develop maps at the state level for these two issues.

b. Create scenes based on your visualization.

c. Based on your scenes, go ahead and use these scenes as images to explain the issues involved.

d. Use these scenes to develop a short video using these two fields.

e. What conclusions do you arrive at?

See Chapter 11, Video Tutorials and Answers to Practice Problems Using Healthcare Datasets in Excel®, for video answers to the practice problems.

References

Bradshaw, P. (n.d.). When to use maps in data visualisation: A great big guide [Blog post]. Retrieved from https://onlinejournalismblog.com/2015/08/24/when-to-use-maps-in-data-visualisation-a-great-big-guide

County Health Rankings and Roadmaps. (n.d.). Explore your snapshot. Retrieved from http://www.countyhealthrankings.org/explore-health-rankings/use-data/exploring-data

Microsoft Office Support. (n.d.). Get started with Power Map. Retrieved from https://support.office.com/en-us/article/get-started-with-power-map-88a28df6-8258-40aa-b5cc-577873fb0f4a

Tableau. (n.d.). *Visual analysis best practices: A guidebook* [White paper]. Retrieved from https://www.tableau.com/learn/whitepapers/tableau-visual-guidebook

USING ANALYSIS OF VARIANCE (ANOVA) IN HEALTHCARE DATASETS TO COMPARE GROUPS AND TEST HYPOTHESES IN EXCEL®

LEARNING OBJECTIVES

- Identify situations where ANOVA test is applicable
- Appreciate the use of ANOVA test in healthcare decision-making
- Create categories of variables in Excel
- Make changes to display of data in preparation for ANOVA test
- Compute confidence interval around mean
- Interpret output from ANOVA test

In this chapter, we use the ANOVA test in Excel to compare three or more groups or categories and test hypotheses about their mean values. The focus in this chapter is on the competency domains of critical thinking, performance management, and problem-solving.

8.1 ANOVA

ANOVA is the test of choice when we wish to determine if the average values for a variable across three or more categories are equal or not (Keller, 2006; Quirk, 2016; SPSS Tutorials, n.d.). For example, in Box 8.1, when length of stay and its relationship across department, urgent stay, interaction of department, and urgent stay is to be assessed, we have three categories that are appropriate for testing using ANOVA.

Throughout the chapter supplemental content is available for the datasets and tutorial videos. Video availability is denoted with an icon. To gain access to these items, please visit the following urls:

Datasets: https://connect.springerpub.com/content/book/978-0-8261-5028-8

⊙ Tutorial Videos: https://connect.springerpub.com/content/book/978-0-8261-5028-8/chapter/ch11

BOX 8.1 ANALYSIS OF VARIANCE AND LENGTH OF STAY AT HOSPITAL

Given escalating healthcare costs across the world, there is continued interest in exploring ways to reduce costs at hospitals while still ensuring that quality standards are adhered to. In order to better understand this issue, a study, exploring the relationship between length of stay of chronic obstructive pulmonary disease (COPD) patients and quality based on observational data post a Six Sigma program, is studied by researchers at a 384-bed medium-sized hospital in the Netherlands (Bisgaard & Does, 2008). These researchers use ANOVA to assess which factors are potentially related to length of stay and which are not. Based on their study, they found that for COPD patients ($n = 143$) there is a significant relationship ($p = 0.015$) between length of stay and being admitted in the pulmonary department rather than the internal medicine department. However, for length of stay of COPD patients and their gender, there was no significant relationship ($p = 0.321$). Lastly, for length of stay of COPD patients who were admitted in an emergency (vs. planned admission), there was no significant relationship ($p = 0.299$). Additional analysis found that COPD patients admitted to the internal medicine department stayed 2.4 days longer than COPD patients admitted to the pulmonary department.

Based on this analysis, given the Six Sigma initiative, the hospital decided to ensure COPD patients are admitted to the pulmonary department and not to the internal medicine department.

In our example of Hospital Consumer Assessment of Healthcare Providers and Systems (HCAHPS) survey for Veterans Administration (VA) facilities (Dataset 3), if we would like to test if the average values of any of the composite measures (e.g., "Understood Care," "Doctor Communication,") categorized by star ratings (one to five stars) are equal, our test of choice is ANOVA. This is the basic test and is also referred to as "ANOVA Single Factor"—the factor in this case that varies is the star rating. We will explore ANOVA using an example.

As can be seen through the boxed research and the proposed example for ANOVA, this analysis lends itself to analyzing the significance of relationships between one variable and another variable that has more than two categories. Viewed thus, the ANOVA extends the *t*-test that was introduced earlier for testing two means. Under ANOVA, we can go ahead and test more than two categories at the same time to find out if the relationship is significant or not. This aids decision-making in a variety of settings such as hospitals if we wish to compare more than two departments on their revenue collections and patient volumes. In other settings, if we wish to explore outcomes or insurance coverage in more than two locations, ANOVA would help us to assess if a significant relationship exists and which of these locations has the significantly favorable outcome or coverage.

8.2 Creating Categories

In order to test for differences of means across three or more categories, we need to have categories to test. In our dataset on HCAHPS survey from VA facilities (Dataset 3), we already have categories of "High" and "Medium" for "Recommend Hospital." Let us create a high, medium, and low categorization of "Rating 9 or 10" using the cutoffs above 75th percentile for high; above 50th percentile for medium; and low if the percentile is below 50th percentile or median. Creating these categories will show us for each facility whether we have a high, medium, or low percentage of patients who gave the facility a "Rating of 9 or 10."

Let us go to our worksheet containing these data and first get the descriptive statistics for "Rating of 9 or 10" to then proceed to establish the cutoffs and categorize this field as high, medium, or low. The easiest way to get these percentiles is to use the Quartile function (=Quartile.Inc) (Figure 8.1). Use this function to establish the 75th percentile (third or upper quartile) and the 50th percentile (second quartile or median). For "Rating of 9 or 10" these are found to be 74 and 68, respectively.

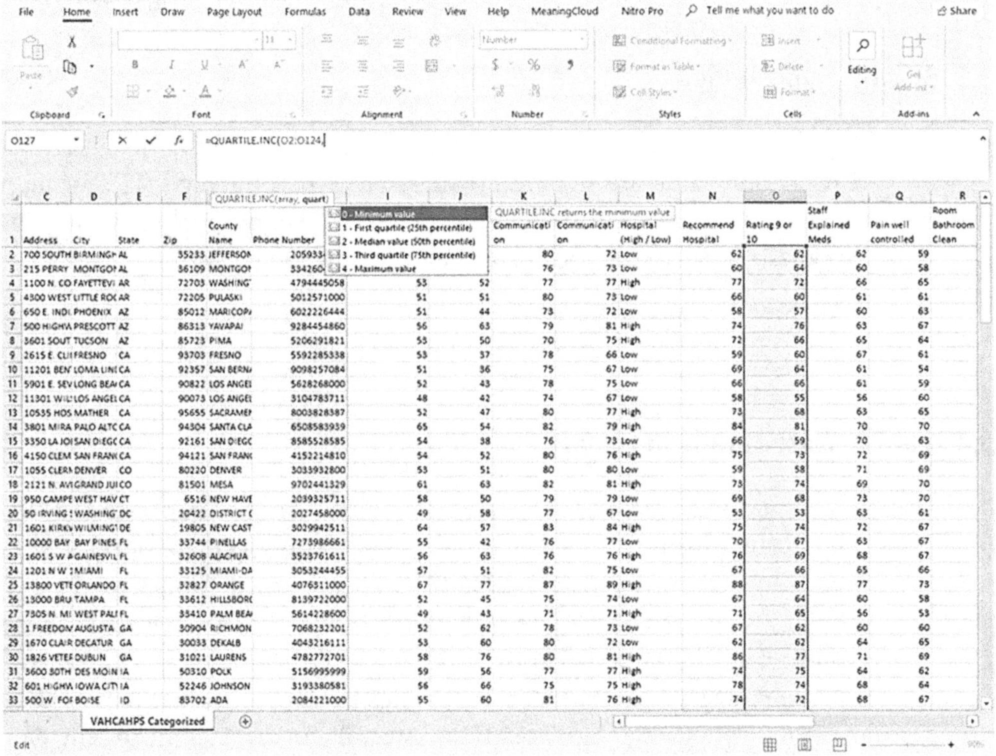

FIGURE 8.1 Creating quartiles for cutoffs.

Tutorial video for Section 8.2 is available by accessing the following url: https://connect .springerpub.com/content/book/978-0-8261-5028-8/chapter/ch11

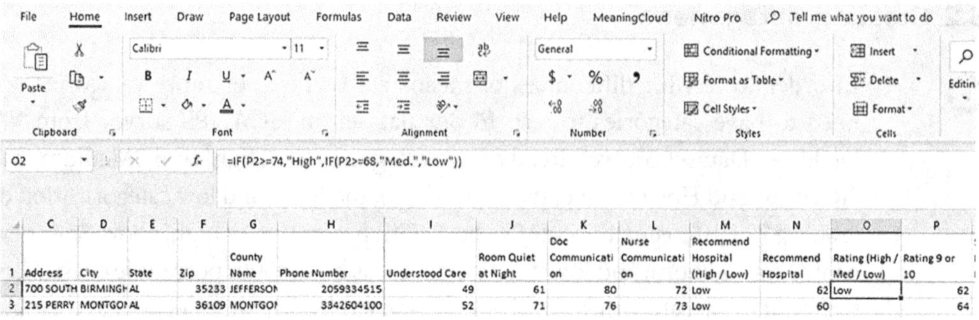

FIGURE 8.2 IF function to create cutoffs.

Now, we will use these cutoffs in an "IF" function to create the categories. First, insert a blank column before the field "Rating of 9 or 10" (Figure 8.2) and label the column as "Rating (High/Med/Low)." In the first blank cell, below the header, we will type in a nested IF function "=IF(P2>=74, "High," IF(P2 ≥ 68, "Med.," "Low"))" that will use the data from "Rating of 9 or 10" and the values for the 50th and 75th percentiles to categorize these data. Once the formula is established in the first cell, click on the square at the bottom of the cell selection and drag and fill the entire column to get the intended categorization.

8.3 Stating Hypotheses

Having established categories, we are now ready to test if the means of "Understood Care" are significantly different across the high (H), medium (M), and low (L) categories of "Rating of 9 or 10." For purposes of testing this hypothesis, we will state the null and alternate hypotheses as:

H_0: $Mean_H$ = $Mean_M$ = $Mean_L$

H_A: $Mean_H$ ≠ $Mean_M$ ≠ $Mean_L$

8.4 Getting Data Ready in Excel

To get started with the ANOVA test, let us first sort our category variable—"Rating High/Med. Low." Next, for purposes of running the ANOVA test in Excel, we need to have our variable that is being tested "Understood Care" in columns for each of the three categories. One way to do so is to go ahead and insert a blank column before "Understood Care" and then cut and paste the entire category and paste this in the empty column. Because the variables are sorted by "Rating High/Med./Low" we will go ahead and copy the data for each of these categories for "Understood Care" and paste it in a separate worksheet in columns labeled with the categories. Go ahead and click and

Tutorial video for Sections 8.3 to 8.5 is available by accessing the following url: https://connect.springerpub.com/content/book/978-0-8261-5028-8/chapter/ch11

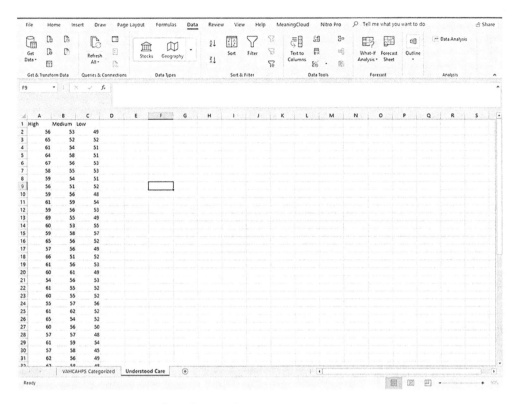

FIGURE 8.3 Organizing data for ANOVA.

create a new worksheet and rename the worksheet "Understood Care." Next, in this new worksheet, label the first three columns as "High," "Medium," and "Low." Go back to your worksheet with the sorted data and copy the sorted data for the "High" category. Click on the "Understood Care" worksheet and paste these data in the column labeled "High." Repeat this process for "Medium" and "Low" (Figure 8.3).

Now, through "Data" on the toolbar, click on "Data Analysis" on the ribbon and scroll and choose "Anova Single Factor" (Figure 8.4). In the "Anova Single Factor" panel that opens (Figure 8.5), go ahead and click the "up arrow" next to "Input range" and then select all three columns of data. Because the sample sizes for the categories (high/medium/low) are not equal, make doubly sure that in each column you have selected all the data. Now make sure to choose "Column" for "Grouped by" and to check "Labels in first row." You have the option to change the alpha level or level of significance of the test. By default, it is 0.05. This is the default 95% level of significance. Finally, you can choose where you want the output of this ANOVA test to go. By default, this goes to a new worksheet.

Before reviewing the ANOVA output, an optional step is to include the confidence interval of "Understood Care" for each of these three categories. We covered confidence interval in Chapter 4 (Setting Bounds for Healthcare Data and Hypothesis Testing Using Excel®) in the section "Setting Bounds on Data." In Figure 8.6, the formulae used for these computations and the output from these formulae are provided. The confidence interval is equal to

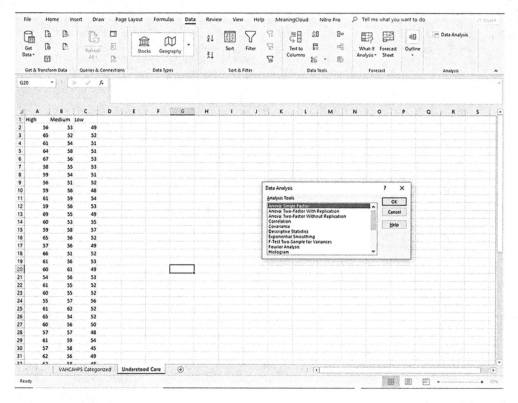

FIGURE 8.4 Choosing ANOVA.

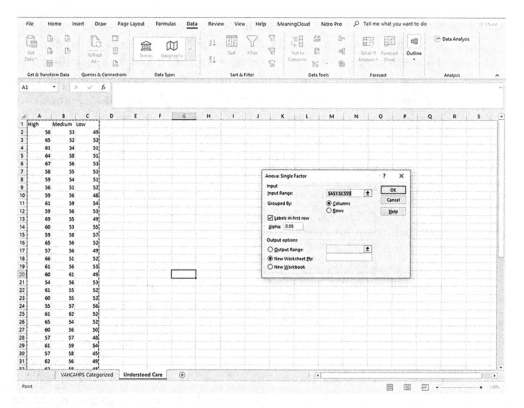

FIGURE 8.5 Selecting data for ANOVA.

=AVERAGE(A2:A55)	=AVERAGE(B2:B55)	=AVERAGE(C2:C55)	Average
=STDEV.S(A2:A33)	=STDEV.S(B2:B38)	=STDEV.S(C2:C55)	Std. Dev.
=A58/SQRT(32)	=B58/SQRT(37)	=C58/SQRT(54)	S.E of Mean
=1.96*A59	=1.96*B59	=1.96*C59	1.96 * S.E of Mean

60.59375	56.37838	51.7037	Average
3.554728	2.680706	2.981893	Std. Dev.
0.628393	0.440705	0.405784	S.E of Mean
1.23165	0.863783	0.795337	1.96 * S.E of Mean

FIGURE 8.6 Mean and standard error of mean.

the Mean ± 1.96* standard error of the mean. Because the ANOVA output already contains the mean, we compute 1.96* standard error of the mean and include this in the ANOVA output.

8.5 Interpreting ANOVA Output

Go to the new worksheet that contains the output of the ANOVA test (Figure 8.7). You will need to resize the columns to see all the output clearly and not as overlapping cells. The first panel contains summary statistics on the variable "Understood Care" for the three groups. This includes the number in the sample (count), the average as well as the variance. The averages for the three groups—high, medium, and low—are very different. This situation is thus a good example of the need to use the ANOVA test to assess the statistical significance of the difference in the means of these three groups. Next, we consider the variance. Any time this variance is very different across groups, there is danger of violating the assumption of homoscedasticity that is required for the ANOVA test. In this example, the variances are different. Unfortunately, there is no simple and easy way to test for homoscedasticity in Excel. So if the variances are not very different, you should be able to undertake ANOVA.

The next panel is the actual output from running the ANOVA test (Figure 8.7). Because this is an ANOVA, the test output reports both the variance between the three categories and within all the pooled categories. In this output, the F-test statistic is reported as well as its probability and critical value. Since the probability is very, very small (3.6E-24), or a decimal followed by 23 zeros, we fail to accept the null hypothesis of no difference in means of "Understood Care" across the three categories. This conclusion is also confirmed by the F-test statistic being much larger than the critical F-value.

Based on this ANOVA analysis of the mean of the variable "Understood Care" across high-, medium-, and low-rated VA facilities, we conclude that

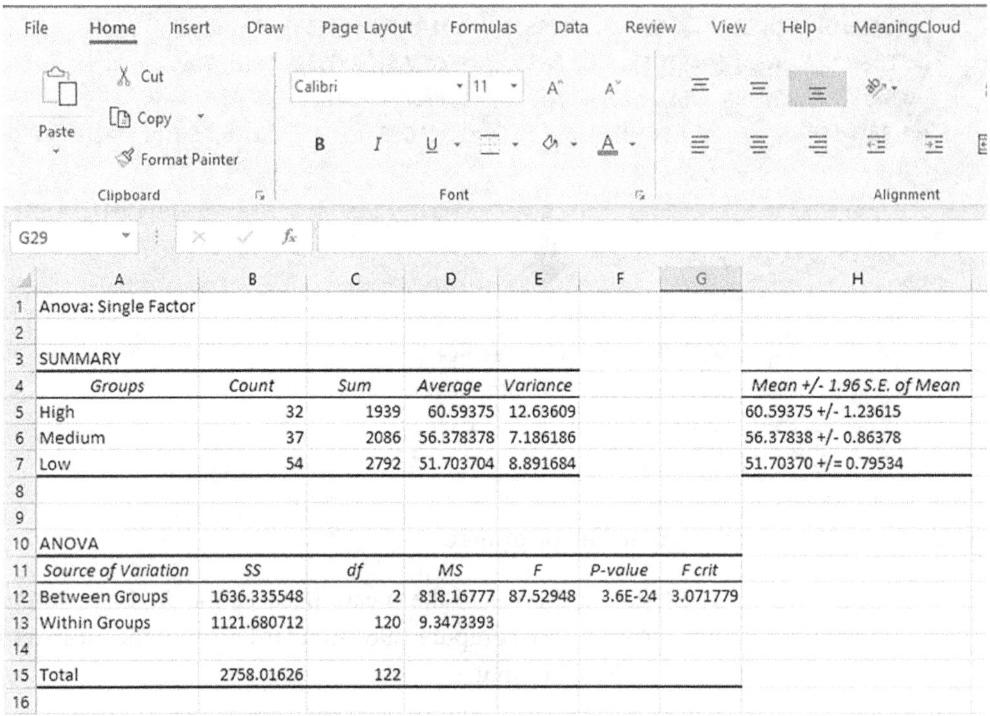

	A	B	C	D	E	F	G	H
1	Anova: Single Factor							
2								
3	SUMMARY							
4	*Groups*	*Count*	*Sum*	*Average*	*Variance*			*Mean +/- 1.96 S.E. of Mean*
5	High	32	1939	60.59375	12.63609			60.59375 +/- 1.23615
6	Medium	37	2086	56.378378	7.186186			56.37838 +/- 0.86378
7	Low	54	2792	51.703704	8.891684			51.70370 +/= 0.79534
8								
9								
10	ANOVA							
11	*Source of Variation*	*SS*	*df*	*MS*	*F*	*P-value*	*F crit*	
12	Between Groups	1636.335548	2	818.16777	87.52948	3.6E-24	3.071779	
13	Within Groups	1121.680712	120	9.3473393				
14								
15	Total	2758.01626	122					
16								

FIGURE 8.7 ANOVA output.

there is a significant difference. This implies that the higher mean value of "Understood Care" (60.59375 ± 1.23615) in high-rated VA facilities is significantly different from the low- and medium-rated VA facilities. Note that with the confidence interval, the true mean value for "Understood Care" in high-rated VA facilities could be as low as 59.3576 or as high as 61.830. Having established this relationship between high-rated VA facilities and "Understood Care" is not by chance, we can then try to understand what happens in high-rated VA facilities that lead to high mean values of "Understood Care" and attempt to replicate it in other VA facilities.

8.6 Competency Development

A study using ANOVA is the subject of Box 8.1. In this study, the researchers are interested in exploring and identifying significant factors that affect length of stay for COPD patients. Based on data collected from the hospital and running ANOVA, they were able to isolate being admitted in the pulmonary department rather than internal medicine department as having a significant relationship with length of stay. Other factors such as gender and being admitted through the emergency department were not found to be significant factors for length of stay. Because there was an ongoing Six Sigma initiative at the hospital, the results of this study rolled directly into ensuring that COPD patients were admitted through the pulmonary department and not the internal medicine department. In ANOVA studies such as this research, pondering over the situation and problem (length of stay of COPD patients) provided the impetus for exploring factors that might be significantly associated with this problem. Having narrowed down on a list of potential factors—at least three—the focus of ANOVA is to test the equality of average values of our dependent variable (length of stay in this case) across these factors. The next step was to collect data on length of stay and these potential factors and then run ANOVA to test for significant factors. Here, identifying the situation and context as well as narrowing down on the problem and potential factors leads to application of skills from the competency domains of critical thinking and problem-solving.

Any time we are testing the equality of a dependent variable across three or more categories, ANOVA is our test of choice. Noting here that if we were testing a dependent variable across two categories, we could use the *t*-test. With our data in Excel, we can use the descriptive statistics routine to identify and develop categories in case these are not already available. With these categories, we are all set to run the ANOVA test in Excel and interpret the ANOVA output. Having already established that for our problem, ANOVA is the test of choice, we make sure that the data setup in Excel is appropriate (three or more categories) and we can then complete the steps for running ANOVA in Excel. These steps, together with the interpretation of results of ANOVA for decision-making provide application of skills from the competency domains of critical thinking and performance management.

In this chapter, identification of situations where the ANOVA test is applicable and making modifications in Excel to run this test leads to development of competency domains of critical thinking and problem-solving. Interpreting the results of the ANOVA test and using it in healthcare decision-making focuses on the competency domains of critical thinking and performance management.

8.7 Summary

Here we extend the testing of means of data from two categories to two or more categories through the ANOVA test. In so doing, we gain a better appreciation of situations where this test can be undertaken. In case categories to test the mean do not already exist in the data, steps to create categories in Excel are provided in this chapter. Finally, interpretation of ANOVA test output informs healthcare decision-making.

8.8 Discussion Questions

8.8.1 Under what situations would you be able to use the ANOVA test? Please describe using an example.

8.8.2 What advantages does the ANOVA test have over a *t*-test? Please explain.

8.8.3 What kinds of decision-making are facilitated through the ANOVA test? Describe using an example.

8.9 Practice Problems

All datasets required for the practice problems are available for download at http://connect.springerpub.com/content/book/978-0-8261-5028-8.

8.9.1 For Dataset 3, which contains HCAHPS survey data from VA facilities, how would you test if there is a difference in mean values for "Doctor Communication" across high/medium/low categories of "Recommend Hospital"?

   a. Define high/medium/low categories for "Recommend Hospital" using the 75th percentile as cutoff for high and the 50th percentile as the cutoff for medium.

   b. State your null and alternate hypotheses.

   c. Run a test to accept or reject your hypotheses. State your test statistics and interpretation of the results.

8.9.2 For Dataset 3, which contains HCAHPS survey data from VA facilities, how would you test if there is a difference in mean values for "Nurse Communication" across high/medium/low categories of "Recommend Hospital"?

   a. Define high/medium/low categories for "Recommend Hospital" using the 75th percentile as cutoff for high and the 50th percentile as the cutoff for medium.

   b. State your null and alternate hypotheses.

   c. Run a test to accept or reject your hypotheses. State your test statistics and interpretation of the results.

8.9.3 For Dataset 12, which contains County Health Rankings, how would you test if there is a difference in mean values for "Physically Unhealthy Days" across high/medium/low categories of "Percent Uninsured?"

   a. Define high/medium/low categories for "Percent Uninsured" using the 75th percentile as cutoff for high and the 50th percentile as the cutoff for medium.

   b. State your null and alternate hypotheses.

   c. Run a test to accept or reject your hypotheses. State your test statistics and interpretation of the results.

8.9.4 For Dataset 12, which contains County Health Rankings, how would you test if there is a difference in mean values for "Mentally Unhealthy Days" across high/medium/low categories of "Percent Uninsured?"

Tutorial videos provided for Practice Problems 8.9.1—8.9.7 can be accessed by accessing the following url: https://connect.springerpub.com/content/book/978-0-8261-5028-8/chapter/ch11

a. Define high/medium/low categories for "Percent Uninsured" using the 75th percentile as cutoff for high and the 50th percentile as the cut off for medium.

b. State your null and alternate hypotheses.

c. Run a test to accept or reject your hypotheses. State your test statistics and interpretation of the results.

8.9.5 For Dataset 10, which contains HCAHPS Summary data for October 2018, how would you test if there is a difference in mean values for "Doctor Communication" across high/medium/low categories of "Recommend Hospital?"

a. Define high/medium/low categories for "Recommend Hospital" using the 75th percentile as cutoff for high and the 50th percentile as the cut off for medium.

b. State your null and alternate hypotheses.

c. Run a test to accept or reject your hypotheses. State your test statistics and interpretation of the results.

8.9.6 For Dataset 10, which contains HCAHPS Summary data for October 2018, how would you test if there is a difference in mean values for "Nurse Communication" across high/medium/low categories of "Recommend Hospital?"

a. Define high/medium/low categories for "Recommend Hospital" using the 75th percentile as cutoff for high and the 50th percentile as the cutoff for medium.

b. State your null and alternate hypotheses.

c. Run a test to accept or reject your hypotheses. State your test statistics and interpretation of the results.

8.9.7 You are working in the Benefits department of an organization. Over the years, there has been this constant crescendo of grumblings from employees about the increase in healthcare insurance premiums for which they are responsible. As the new enrollment season rolls around, you set out to investigate this relationship to see if these rising premiums have impacted the number of people with employer-provided coverage. Use Dataset 9 to investigate if there is a statistical difference in mean values of "People with employer coverage 2015" across high/medium/low categories of "Average Annual Growth in Family Premium for Employer Coverage 2010–2015."

a. Define high/medium/low categories for "Average Annual Growth in Family Premium for Employer Coverage 2010–2015" using the 75th percentile as cutoff for high and the 50th percentile as the cutoff for medium.

      b. State your null and alternate hypotheses.

      c. Run a test to accept or reject your hypotheses. State your test statistics and interpretation of the results.

      d. What implications do you draw from this test for employer coverage and the growth in family premium?

See Chapter 11, Video Tutorials and Answers to Practice Problems Using Healthcare Datasets in Excel®, for video answers to the practice problems.

References

Bisgaard, S., & Does, R. J. M. M. (2008). Quality quandaries: Health care quality—Reducing the length of stay at a hospital. *Quality Engineering, 21*(1), 117–131. doi:10.1080/08982110802529612

Keller, D. K. (2006). *The tao of statistics: A path to understanding (with no math).* Thousand Oaks, CA: Sage Publications.

Quirk, T. J. (2016). *Excel 2016 for health services management statistics: A guide to solving practical problems.* New York, NY: Springer.

SPSS Tutorials. (n.d.). ANOVA—Simple introduction. Retrieved from https://www.spss-tutorials.com/anova-what-is-it

9

TEXT ANALYSIS OF HEALTHCARE DATA USING MEANINGCLOUD ADD-IN IN EXCEL®

LEARNING OBJECTIVES

- Appreciate the use of social media in healthcare research
- Use MeaningCloud Add-in in Excel
- Use key questions to guide qualitative analysis
- Apply text categorization using classification models
- Undertake sentiment analysis using general and customized models
- Analyze textual data using topic extraction to identify themes
- Analyze textual data using text clustering
- Apply pivot tables and charts to analyzed textual data
- Use analyzed textual data to aid healthcare decision-making

In this chapter, we use the MeaningCloud Add-In in Excel to perform several types of qualitative analysis. A hypothetical example is used for text classification, sentiment analysis, topic extraction, and text clustering. The focus of this chapter is on the competency domains of critical thinking, information management, and problem-solving.

Throughout the chapter supplemental content is available for the datasets and tutorial videos. Video availability is denoted with an icon. To gain access to these items, please visit the following urls:

Datasets: https://connect.springerpub.com/content/book/978-0-8261-5028-8

⊙ Tutorial Videos: https://connect.springerpub.com/content/book/978-0-8261-5028-8/chapter/ch11

BOX 9.1 SOCIAL MEDIA AND HEALTHCARE

Social media has been witnessing an exponential growth. In early 2018, a Pew Research study (Smith & Anderson, 2018) found that 68% of adults used Facebook and between 22% and 35% of adults were users of WhatsApp, Twitter, LinkedIn, Snapchat, Pinterest, and Instagram. With increasing proliferation of mobile devices, it is becoming even easier to access social media through smartphones and tablets. With this kind of growth and reach, it is not surprising that the use of social media sites such as Twitter, Facebook, and LinkedIn for healthcare research (Azer, 2017) and for health behavior intervention (Arigo, Pagoto, Carter-Harris, Lillie, & Nebeker, 2018) is growing. This growth is being fueled not just by consumers but also the healthcare industry itself. In a survey of stakeholders from healthcare systems, approximately three-fourths report that their organizations use social media for care delivery initiatives such as chronic disease management, health behavior promotion, and emotional support (Volpp & Mohta, 2017).

In a systematic review of 22 articles on the use of social media for healthcare research and intervention (Smailhodzic, Hooijsma, Boonstra, & Langley, 2016), researchers concluded that social media has the following effects on patients:

- Improved self-management and control
- Improved psychological well-being
- Improved subjective well-being
- Diminished subjective well-being
- Addiction to social media
- Loss of privacy
- Targeted for promotions

These researchers also concluded from this review that social media has several important effects on the patient–provider relationship too— more equal communication, increased switching of providers, harmonious relationship, and suboptimal relationship. Within these effects on patients as well as the patient–provider relationship, it is not surprising to note that at times contradictory effects from different studies are found as well as a recognition that social media can be a double-edged sword.

In a nod to wearable technology and how that is providing a boost to the use of social media to monitor patient care, social media has been acknowledged as the new "vital" sign (Young, 2018).

While acknowledging the growth in the use of social media, several researchers are also quick to point out the still unresolved challenges

(continued)

> **BOX 9.1** (*continued*)
>
> of confidentiality, privacy, informed consent, as well as ethical issues (Arigo et al., 2018; Azer, 2017; Young, 2018). Given the uneven growth in social media and because of disparities in access, there is unrealized potential with vulnerable populations (Smith & Smith, 2015).

9.1 Qualitative Data in Healthcare

The growth in the use of social media for healthcare research and intervention (see Box 9.1) has opened the veritable floodgates of qualitative data that is now available for analysis and decision-making. Because social media is ubiquitous in its growing presence in the healthcare industry for health behavior interventions, monitoring patient data occasioned by wearable technology, and for research and feedback, we have unique access to unfiltered comments and thoughts of patients, providers, and other stakeholders. In attempting to mine this qualitative data, admittedly we need to be sensitive to the privacy, confidentiality, and ethical challenges that social media brings.

Qualitative data from social media as well as surveys and interviews contain rich information. Lest this rich information remain untapped and unused, we need to have tools and techniques to tap into these data and use them for decision-making. Because much of these qualitative data pertain to research questions, health interventions, or feedback, they lend themselves to decision-making. There is a range of free to very expensive and sophisticated qualitative analysis software that can be used to analyze qualitative data. In this chapter, we focus on the use of an Add-in to Excel that provides an alternative approach within Excel to manage simple analysis of qualitative data.

9.2 Qualitative Analysis and Excel

Frequent users of Excel will recognize that text or qualitative analysis is not the first thing that comes to mind in their use of Excel. Since Excel is so ubiquitously identified with quantitative analysis, it is a far stretch to think of using Excel to perform any qualitative analysis. Through the MeaningCloud Add-in, hopefully we can shatter this myth.

Qualitative analysis shares a key feature with quantitative analysis—they are both guided by the research question that needs to be answered before we consider what methods we bring to bear on the analysis. Thus, our research question would guide the design of research as well as the collection and analysis of data.

There are several specialized software that undertake very sophisticated kinds of qualitative and related analyses. Through the MeaningCloud Add-in in Excel, we are trading the sophistication for a limited set of qualitative analyses that can be performed within the Excel environment. The basic idea that is emphasized using this Add-in is to be able to analyze open-ended responses that are included in surveys. By using this Add-in, we can undertake text classification, sentiment analysis, topic extraction, and text clustering. In the sections mentioned subsequently, we will use sample textual data to explore how these analyses are accomplished through the MeaningCloud Add-in.

9.3 MeaningCloud Add-In

The MeaningCloud Add-in can be downloaded from the MeaningCloud website (www.meaningcloud.com/developer/excel-addin/doc/download-install). This is a free Add-in that installs in Excel and is added to the Toolbar (Figure 9.1). Once installed, you need to register your Add-in and are provided a license key to activate the analytic features.

Once you have installed and activated MeaningCloud Add-in in Excel, you are now ready to get down to performing qualitative analyses with the built-in analytical features in this Add-in. Typically, the data with which you will be working would be open-ended responses to surveys or any structured textual response that you have. The example we use to explore the analytical features in this Add-in, Dataset 14, is based on hypothetical data on patient experiences at a hospital. Data such as these are collected based on responses by patients or caregivers after a visit to a hospital. There could be many such responses that might be available by individual respondents. In our example, there are 20 responses in one column and a respondent ID in one column.

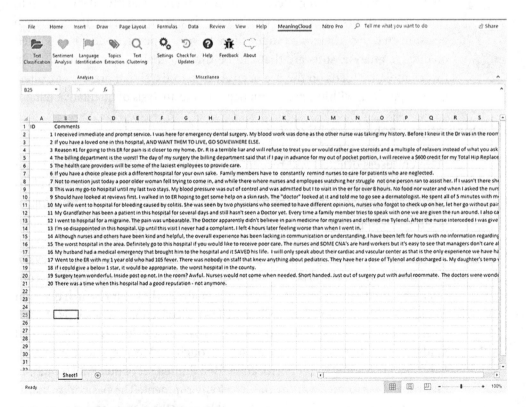

FIGURE 9.1 MeaningCloud Add-in.

The collection of patient experiences is usually guided by trying to understand how satisfied patients are with their experiences in the hospital and, if there are suggestions for improvement, how best to respond to them. A quick scan of these responses shows that there were more patients and caregivers who were unhappy with the care that they received at the hospital. However, rather than being limited to these broad generalizations, we would like to analyze and possibly categorize these responses. Categorization can be done through coding or classification and is a key feature of qualitative analysis (Stake, 2010).

9.4 Text Classification

Once we are in the worksheet with text responses, we can go ahead and click on "MeaningCloud" in the toolbar (Figure 9.1). Once the Add-in is invoked, the ribbon shows us the analysis options—the first of which is "Text Classification." A new panel (Figure 9.2) opens that will be used to identify our text responses or the data that is to be analyzed. We go ahead and click on the icon next to "Select cells with text to analyze" and choose the column of text responses—all 20 rows in this column. Next, we check, "I want to specify IDs" and click the icon next to "Select cell with the IDs column." Note that for the IDs you need to select just one cell (any cell) in the ID column and not the entire column of IDs.

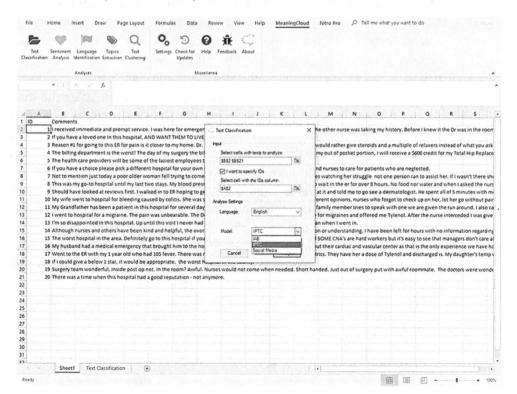

FIGURE 9.2 Text classification using MeaningCloud Add-in.

Tutorial video for Section 9.4 is available by accessing the following url: https://connect .springerpub.com/content/book/978-0-8261-5028-8/chapter/ch11

In the analysis section of this panel, for the model we have three choices from which to choose. These models contain present classifications that can be applied to our text that needs to be analyzed. These three models represent the following (MeaningCloud, n.d.):

1. IAB (Interactive Advertising Bureau)—a standard classification used in the advertising industry
2. IPTC (International Press Telecommunications Council)—a standard classification used in the news media
3. Social Media—a standard classification used in social media

Depending on your source of text response as well as based on your research question, you would choose one of these three models to be used for classification of your text responses. Among these three models, IPTC is the most extensive with over 1,400 categories. We go ahead and choose IPTC as our model to be used for classification of text responses and then click "Ok."

The chosen model is run and a new worksheet with the analyzed text as well as categorization based on the model chosen is developed (Figure 9.3). This output shows the categorization, as well as rank and relevance of these categories. Because the text responses have been analyzed, we can also include this analysis in a pivot chart and better represent the analysis. To do so, from your worksheet with the analyzed text, click on "Insert" in the toolbar and click on "Pivot Chart" (Figure 9.4). Once the panel for "Pivot Chart" opens, make sure that your entire data table is selected and click "Ok."

In a new worksheet, a pivot table and chart are revealed. Using the steps identified in sections "Using Pivot Tables" and "Pivot Charts" of Chapter 3 (Identifying, Categorizing, and Presenting Healthcare Data Using Excel®) we can go ahead and summarize the information from the fields in a pivot table and pivot chart. For this example, we can drag "Labels" and "Relevance" from the Field List to "Values" and "ID" to "Rows" to get a simple pivot chart (Figure 9.5). Depending on the research question, additional summarization of results through pivot tables and pivot charts can be undertaken.

Note that for this example, we used the preset models for our categorization. Advanced users can use unique characteristics of their data and research question to create their own models for categorization.

9.5 Sentiment Analysis

Next, we move on to consider sentiment analysis. Sentiment analysis is used to assess the kinds of sentiments that are conveyed by the text responses. These

---

Tutorial video for Section 9.5 is available by accessing the following url: https://connect .springerpub.com/content/book/978-0-8261-5028-8/chapter/ch11

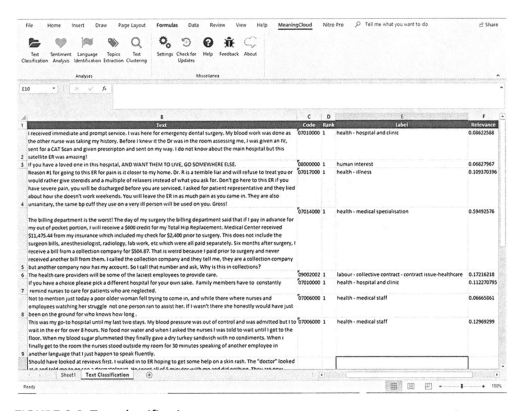

FIGURE 9.3 Text classification output.

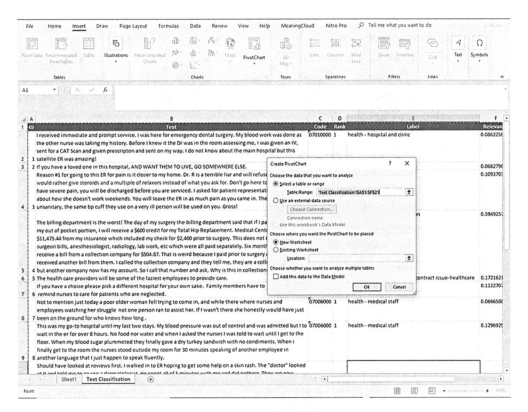

FIGURE 9.4 Inserting pivot chart for text classification output.

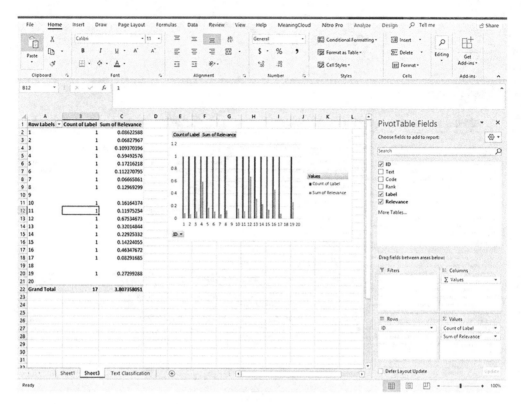

FIGURE 9.5 Pivot chart for text classification output.

general sentiments conveyed through the text responses are categorized as being positive, negative, or neutral as well as whether they convey agreement or disagreement. The general model for sentiment analysis can also be customized based on our data to be more specific to the research question and analysis proposed.

Go back to your original worksheet containing the 20 test responses and the IDs. Click on "MeaningCloud" in the toolbar and now choose "Sentiment Analysis." The panel for "Sentiment Analysis" opens and we can go ahead and identify our input data as well as "ID" as described (mentioned previously) for Text Classification (Figure 9.6).

The output for sentiment analysis appears in two new worksheets—global sentiment analysis (Figure 9.7) and topic sentiment analysis. Because the global level provides overall sentiments, we will focus on the global level. In order to use the output from topic sentiment analysis, customization of the analysis is recommended.

In the first analysis column, "Polarity," the text responses are categorized as being positive, negative, or neutral and the second column relates these responses to agreement. Because this is based on a general model, it appears that, since most responses are not flattering to the hospital, this is the reference frame for this general analysis. The last column provides a conclusion on the use of irony in the response.

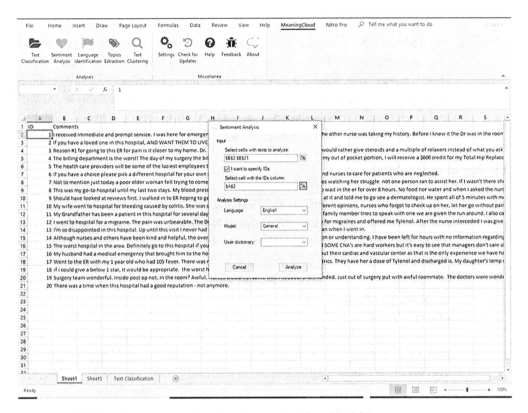

FIGURE 9.6 Sentiment analysis using MeaningCloud Add-in.

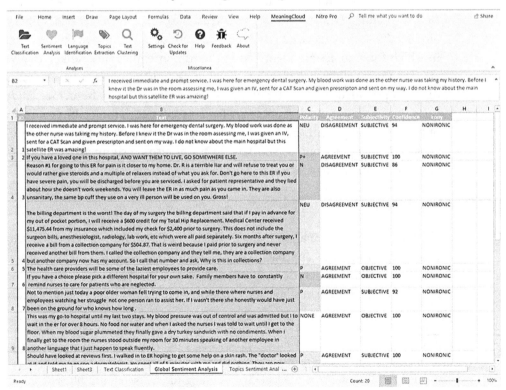

FIGURE 9.7 Output for global sentiment analysis.

This sentiment analysis is again an attempt to categorize and identify themes and patterns underlying the data. A closer reading of the text responses akin to "living with the data" (Minichiello & Kottler, 2010) would lead to these themes. Here the MeaningCloud Add-in attempts to do a preliminary identification of themes related to sentiments in the text response using a general model. As with text classification, customization can be used to fine-tune sentiment analysis and the output can also be summarized through pivot tables and pivot charts.

9.6 Topic Extraction

Now we move on to consider the next analysis—Topic Extraction. Under this analysis, the text responses are analyzed to assess topics that are embedded in the responses. As with other analyses, this again continues the categorization of responses around topics in order to identify themes and patterns that emerge from the data. Within MeaningCloud, it is possible to customize and use your own models to identify topics. Here we are using the general model to identify topics.

Continuing with the sheet containing the original 20 text responses, we click on "MeaningCloud" in the toolbar and now choose "Topic Extraction." The panel for Topic Extraction is very similar to the previous two analyses that were just done, and we go ahead and identify the data selection as well as the ID field and click "Ok."

The output for Topic Extraction is on a new worksheet (Figure 9.8). For each respondent (ID), topics are extracted as a specific form (service, surgery, blood, etc.) and categorized as either a concept or entity. Based on the order in which these topics are identified in the response, these are ranked to give an idea about saliency of mention. Further categorization of these extracted topics is provided through typology as well as from which branch of study this topic comes. In the last column of analysis, for each topic, the frequency of the topic being mentioned in the text response for each respondent is provided. This output from Topic Extraction can also be summarized through pivot tables and pivot charts.

9.7 Text Clustering

The final approach to analysis using the MeaningCloud Add-in is through text clustering. Under this approach, data responses are analyzed for words and categories around which the responses cluster. For instance, if in responding to patient experiences in a hospital, the word "bills" or "surgery" is repeatedly

---

Tutorial video for Section 9.6 is available by accessing the following url: https://connect .springerpub.com/content/book/978-0-8261-5028-8/chapter/ch11

Tutorial video for Section 9.7 is available by accessing the following url: https://connect .springerpub.com/content/book/978-0-8261-5028-8/chapter/ch11

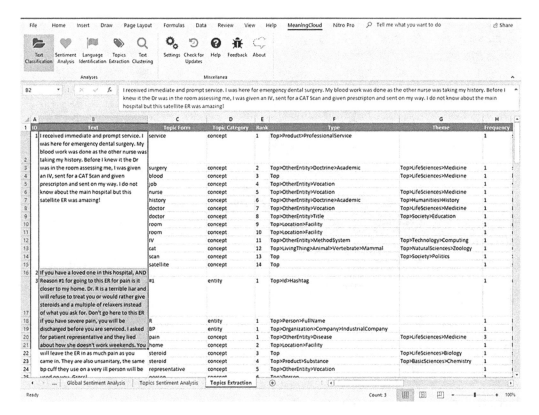

FIGURE 9.8 Output for topics extraction.

brought up, this is identified as a cluster and the size of the cluster represents the number of times that this word was brought up. Within this Add-in, there are two approaches to text clustering (Figure 9.9)—topic modeling and document grouping. As before, we can access our original data and through the toolbar access "Text Clustering." In the interface, after identifying your data, you get to choose the mode or approach to text clustering. In addition, if there are specific words that you choose not to include in the text clustering, these can be added as "Stop Words." In Figure 9.9, the word "I" has been identified as "Stop Word" such that it is not used for clustering.

9.7.1 Topic Modeling

Under the topic "Modeling approach to text clustering," words within the text responses are used for clustering across the text responses (Figure 9.10). The frequency of these words across responses is the basis for the cluster size and the cluster size is used for ranking. If we consider the output, the column "Cluster" includes the specific occurrence of this word in the response, while the cluster size refers to the overall frequency of this word across all responses. Thus, across all responses, "hospital" has the largest cluster size and the largest rank.

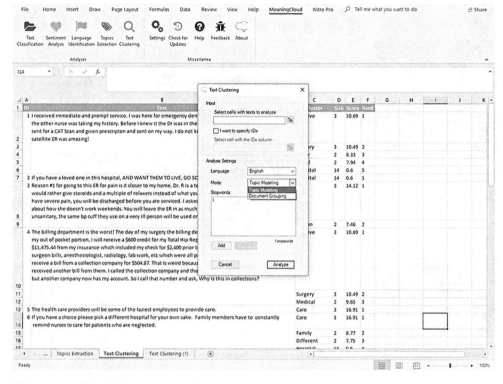

FIGURE 9.9 Interface for text clustering.

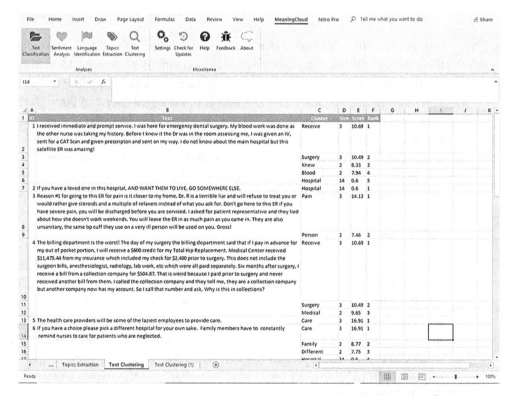

FIGURE 9.10 Output for text clustering: Topic modeling.

This output on text clustering under topic "Modeling approach to text clustering" is summarized using pivot charts (Figure 9.11). Here the ranks and clusters are summarized to show how the words used by respondents cluster across responses and what is the saliency of their clustering.

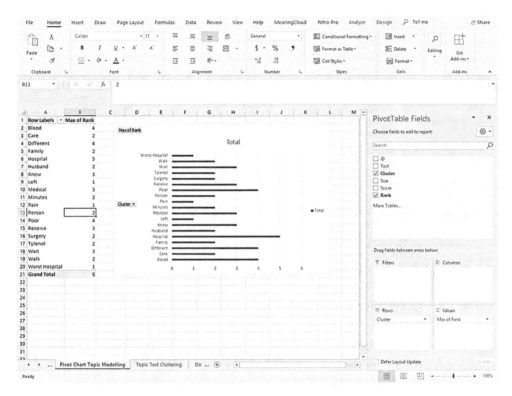

FIGURE 9.11 Topic modeling pivot chart.

9.7.2 Document Grouping

The second approach to text clustering embedded in the interface is document grouping. Under this approach, instead of the actual words used in the responses, here the key ideas in the responses are used for clustering (Figure 9.12). Thus, ideas used for clustering include care, communication, and awful/wonderful. These ideas and the clusters based on their occurrence in the responses are used for cluster size computation. Here, pain, bill, awful/wonderful (contradictory experiences) are among the larger effect sizes.

Again, this output can be summarized through pivot charts to provide a visualization of the clustering. As with the approaches to analysis, customization of the analysis will lead to better analysis rather than through the use of general models.

Through the MeaningCloud Add-in, several approaches to preliminary qualitative text analysis have been shown. Based on the research question

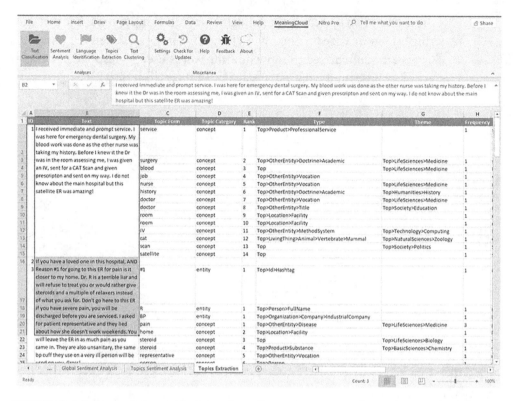

FIGURE 9.12 Output for text clustering: Document grouping.

and data, a determination can be made as to the suitability of one or more approaches. In case more sophisticated qualitative analysis is required, the use of stand-alone qualitative analysis software is recommended.

9.8 Competency Development

The growing role and influence of social media by patients as well as healthcare organizations for healthcare delivery and research are the subject of Box 9.1. Social media opens an interesting facet of data—qualitative or textual—with which we do not interact so frequently and therefore have limited tools and methods to deploy in analyzing these data. Here the ability to start with a problem or issue and develop a framework or model where qualitative data may provide answers and aid decision-making helps to work through the competency domains of information management and problem-solving.

Once we have a question or issues to which qualitative data (through social media or interviews and open-ended responses on surveys) may provide answers, we still need to be able to make sense of the data through focused analysis. Within Excel, the MeaningCloud Add-in provides this capability to undertake initial qualitative analysis. This initial qualitative analysis encompasses four approaches—text classification, sentiment analysis, topic extraction, and text clustering. The choice of one or more of these approaches to qualitative analysis is again based on the question or issues that the data are supposed to answer. Within these approaches, as we gain familiarity with these approaches, we can then either use the provided models for classifications or develop our own models to customize the classification of qualitative data. Using the research question to guide both the choice of qualitative data and the choice of one of the four approaches to qualitative analysis, and choosing between available models or creating our own model for classification in the MeaningCloud Add-in, leads to application of skills from the competency domains of critical thinking and information management.

In this chapter, appreciation of the role of social media and textual data for healthcare decision-making leads to development of information management and problem-solving competency domains. Next, the use of MeaningCloud Add-in in Excel and its suite of analytical modules focuses on critical thinking and information management competency domains.

9.9 Summary

There are several sources of qualitative or textual data. A growing source of such data is from social media as well as open-ended responses on surveys and interviews. By using the MeaningCloud Add-in in Excel, we use qualitative data in Excel for focused analysis using the suite of analytical modules. The analyses include text categorization, sentiment analysis, topic extraction, and text clustering based on standard and customizable models. Results of these analyses are then used in pivot tables and charts for data display. Analyses of qualitative data through the MeaningCloud Add-in aid the use of such data for healthcare decision-making.

9.10 Discussion Questions

9.10.1 Do you think that the use of social media in healthcare research and intervention is a good thing? Why or why not?

9.10.2 Do you think that qualitative analysis has a role to play in healthcare decision-making? Why or why not?

9.10.3 In using Excel for qualitative analysis, is there any loss in data or meaning? How?

9.11 Practice Problems

All datasets required for the practice problems are available for download at http://connect.springerpub.com/content/book/978-0-8261-5028-8.

9.11.1 Use Dataset 15. In this file, there are 12 patient reviews of a visit to a doctor's office. You are an analyst working at this office and are

Tutorial videos provided for Practice Problems 9.11.1—9.11.4 can be accessed by accessing the following url: https://connect.springerpub.com/content/book/978-0-8261-5028-8/chapter/ch11

tasked with analyzing and presenting the data. To undertake your analysis, use the MeaningCloud Add-in in Excel to do the following analyses:

a. Text classification

b. Sentiment analysis

c. Topic extraction, and

d. Text clustering

Wherever appropriate, summarize your analysis using pivot charts. Which of these approaches to qualitative analysis helps you the most to analyze patient reviews? Why?

9.11.2 Use Dataset 16. In this file, there are 12 patient reviews of interaction with nurses during a visit to a doctor's office. You are an analyst working at this office and are tasked with analyzing and presenting the data. To undertake your analysis, use the MeaningCloud Add-in in Excel to do the following analyses:

a. Text classification

b. Sentiment analysis

c. Topic extraction, and

d. Text clustering

Wherever appropriate, summarize your analysis using pivot charts. Which of these approaches to qualitative analysis helps you the most to analyze patient reviews? Why?

9.11.3 You have just been handed these patient reviews of a nursing home (Dataset 17). Use the MeaningCloud Add-in in Excel to classify text and identify topics from these reviews.

a. How would you start your analysis and what approach(es) to analysis will you adopt? Why?

b. Prepare a summary based on your analysis, including appropriate charts and figures.

9.11.4 You have just been handed these patient reviews of a dentist (Dataset 18). Use the MeaningCloud Add-in in Excel to undertake analysis of these reviews to identify sentiments expressed by patients and caregivers.

a. How would you start your analysis and what approach(es) to analysis will you adopt? Why?

b. Prepare a summary based on your analysis, including appropriate charts and figures.

See Chapter 11, Video Tutorials and Answers to Practice Problems Using Healthcare Datasets in Excel®, for video answers to the practice problems.

References

Arigo, D., Pagoto, S., Carter-Harris, L., Lillie, S. E., & Nebeker, C. (2018). Using social media for health research: Methodological and ethical considerations for recruitment and intervention delivery. *Digital Health, 4*. doi:10.1177/2055207618771757

Azer, S. A. (2017). Social media channels in health care research and rising ethical issues. *American Medical Association Journal of Ethics, 19*(11), 1061–1069. doi:10.1001/journalofethics.2017.19.11.peer1-1711

MeaningCloud. (n.d.). MeaningCloud for Excel. Retrieved from https://www.meaningcloud.com/developer/excel-addin/doc/3.3/text-classification

Minichiello, V., & Kottler, J. A. (2010). *Qualitative journeys: Student and mentor experiences with research*. Thousand Oaks, CA: Sage Publications.

Smailhodzic, E., Hooijsma, W., Boonstra, A., & Langley, D. J. (2016). Social media use in healthcare: A systematic review of effects on patients and on their relationship with healthcare professionals. *BMC Health Services Research, 16*(1). doi:10.1186/s12913-016-1691-0

Smith, A., & Anderson, M. (2018, March 1). Social media use 2018. *Pew Research Center*. Retrieved from https://www.pewinternet.org/2018/03/01/social-media-use-in-2018

Smith, B. G., & Smith, S. B. (2015). *Engaging health: Health research and policymaking in the social media sphere*. Washington, DC: AcademyHealth. Retrieved from https://www.academyhealth.org/sites/default/files/AH_Translation%20Engaging%20Health%20Social%20Media%20Sphere.pdf

Stake, R. E. (2010). *Qualitative research: Studying how things work*. New York, NY: Guilford Press.

Volpp, K. G., & Mohta, N. S. (2017). *Social networks to improve patient health* [Insights Report]. Retrieved from https://cdn2.hubspot.net/hubfs/558940/Social%20Networks%20to%20Improve%20Patient%20Health.pdf?__hstc=23193637.bd17a44857c41a5dbfc9d2d1311871ed.1551221557485.1551466530514.1551472569586.4&__hssc=23193637.1.1553991234172&__hsfp=592281695&hsCtaTracking=481f608d-1c97-46ae-b84c-f8363849a161%7C39b7024d-0af2-4424-a021-1a63b42a9c49

Young, S. D. (2018). Social media as a new vital sign: Commentary. *Journal of Medical Internet Research, 20*(4), e161. doi:10.2196/jmir.8563

10

SAMPLING AND RESEARCH DESIGN USING HEALTHCARE DATA IN EXCEL®

LEARNING OBJECTIVES

- Appreciate changes in healthcare and the need for research to evolve
- Use questions and problems as the starting point for research
- Understand the broad categories of random and nonrandom sampling
- Use Excel for generating samples
- Describe the three key elements of research design
- Appreciate the different methods used for research

In this chapter, we go through a brief review of common sampling and research designs. Examples in Excel are used to describe the process of sampling under the different approaches and considerations in hypothesis testing and issues of generalizability from sample to population. The focus of this chapter is on the competency domains of critical thinking and problem-solving.

10.1 Research Driven by Questions

The Agency for Healthcare Research and Quality (AHRQ) Report "Using Rapid-Cycle Research to Reach Goals: Awareness, Assessment, Adaptation, Acceleration" (Johnson, Gustafson, Ewigman, Provost, & Roper, 2015)—see Box 10.1—highlights how research in practice settings has to evolve to keep pace with the rapid changes in healthcare. To those changes, one may

---

Throughout the chapter supplemental content is available for the datasets and tutorial videos. Video availability is denoted with an icon. To gain access to these items, please visit the following urls:

Datasets: https://connect.springerpub.com/content/book/978-0-8261-5028-8

⊙ Tutorial Videos: https://connect.springerpub.com/content/book/978-0-8261-5028-8/chapter/ch11

BOX 10.1 RAPID-CYCLE RESEARCH

In 2015, the Agency for Healthcare Research and Quality (AHRQ) practice-based research network (PBRN) disseminated a commissioned report entitled "Using Rapid-Cycle Research to Reach Goals: Awareness, Assessment, Adaptation, Acceleration" (Johnson et al., 2015). This report is in the public domain and makes a strong case for research design to evolve with changes in healthcare delivery such as horizontal and vertical integration. At the same time, such changes in research design will help to address quality improvement and implementation of interventions by hastening the pace of research to actionable insights. This is the backdrop to rapid-cycle research and an overview of this process is provided here. The content here has been adapted from the AHRQ report cited previously.

A working definition of Rapid-Cycle Research (RCR) provided in this report is "process by which practical problems are identified and addressed using analysis methods that are incremental and contextually informed" (Johnson et al., 2015, p. iv) The RCR consists of six phases (see Figure 10.1) and several steps and processes.

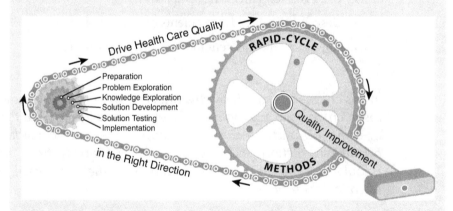

FIGURE 10.1 Rapid-cycle research framework.
SOURCE: Johnson, K., Gustafson, D., Ewigman, B., Provost, L., & Roper, R. (2015). *Using rapid-cycle research to reach goals: Awareness, assessment, adaptation, acceleration* (AHRQ Publication No. 15-0036). Rockville, MD: Agency for Healthcare Research and Quality. Retrieved from https://pbrn.ahrq.gov/sites/default/files/docs/page/AHRQPBRNFinalRapidCycleResearchGuidanceDocument.pdf

Six Phases of RCR

Phase 1: Preparation—Identifying stakeholders (champions and opponents) and understanding their perspectives.

(continued)

BOX 10.1 (*continued*)

Phase 2: Problem exploration—Understanding prioritized problems to solve. Four tools suggested to accomplish a deeper dive into the problem are the following:

a. Walk through—To understand the problem from the client's perspective

b. Nominal group technique—To engage experts to understand possible causes of the problem

c. Critical incident technique—To use the client's description of the problem to identify causes and look for solutions

d. Dialogue—To use shared perspectives from clients and experts to arrive at a common understanding of the problem

Phase 3: Knowledge exploration—Exploring the different facets of the problem through four steps:

a. Characterize the problem in a general way

b. Identify other industries with this general problem

c. Identify industry leaders that have best addressed the problem

d. Identify process or activities that differentiate industry leaders from others

Phase 4: Solution development—Identify the simplest possible solution by applying "ideal design" engineering process.

Phase 5: Solution testing—Determining if identified solutions work through pilot testing. There the testing design and method are determined by question(s) to be answered. (Some potential designs and methods are reviewed briefly here and there are more details as well as real-world examples of each of these in the AHRQ report.)

a. Time series—This design helps to sequence the intervention preceding change/solution. Repeated measures in a time series further increase our confidence in results.

b. Point-of-care randomized control trial—Here, the randomization occurs at the point of delivery of care and helps to address concerns with bias in selection of respondents for intervention.

c. Factorial design—This design helps to compare the effect of several interventions at the same time.

d. Stepped wedge design—This is a form of clustered randomized control trials where the interventions are gradually phased in and eventually every cluster receives the intervention.

(*continued*)

> ### BOX 10.1 (*continued*)
>
> e. Adaptive trial design—This design has planned adaptations that are triggered by end points or certain findings.
>
> Phase 6: Implementation and dissemination—In this phase, resources are identified to scale-up solution and address implementation issues.
>
> Source: Adapted from Johnson, K., Gustafson, D., Ewigman, B., Provost, L., & Roper, R. (2015). *Using rapid-cycle research to reach goals: Awareness, assessment, adaptation, acceleration* (AHRQ Publication No. 15-0036). Rockville, MD: Agency for Healthcare Research and Quality. Retrieved from https://pbrn.ahrq.gov/sites/default/files/docs/page/AHRQPBRNFinalRapidCycleResearchGuidance Document.pdf

also add the deluge of data that we have and how our research designs and methods can take cognizance of these issues. In this backdrop, questions or problems that are identified are the foundations for then designing a methodologically sound study.

For research, the starting point is always the research question (Singleton & Straits, 2010). This is the basis for informing the entire research process from the framing of the research question, through design of instruments, sampling, data collection, analysis, and interpretation. There is a definite structuring of this process to ensure that rigorous research is undertaken through all steps and that we have robust results in which we are confident. There are several textbooks such as *Investigating the Social World* (Schutt, 2015) and *Approaches to Social Research* (Singleton & Straits, 2010) that provide a very detailed explanation of the intricacies of this whole process. For our purposes, to the extent that hypothesis testing and analysis are influenced by key elements of sampling and research design, an overview and appreciation of these issues are provided here.

10.2 Sampling

As alluded to in Chapter 4, Setting Bounds for Healthcare Data and Hypothesis Testing Using Excel®, whenever we do hypothesis testing, we do it in the context of results from our sample and how they compare to population values. For most studies, since the costs of collecting data from all members of the population that the study is about would be prohibitive, we invariably rely on collecting data from a subset or sample of the population. With data collection and analysis predicated on how good a subset or sample of the population is, this impacts our ability to generalize the results from our sample study to the population that this study covers.

Broadly, there are two approaches to sampling—probability and nonprobability. Let us consider these two approaches and the common sampling designs under each of these approaches (Schutt, 2015; Singleton & Straits, 2010).

10.3 Probability Sampling

Under probability sampling, the chance of an element or member of this population being selected in the sample is known prior to the study and is nonzero, meaning that each element has a known probability of being selected in the sample and that this probability is greater than zero—since a zero probability implies no chance of selection. There are four major approaches to probability sampling that we will use as examples to describe probability sampling in Excel.

The example that we have in Excel (Dataset 19) covers all the 3,191 counties and county equivalents in the United States and thus is the population. We will use this population to describe the common probabilistic sampling designs.

10.3.1 Simple Random Sampling

Sample selection under simple random sampling is based purely on chance and is random—random in a statistical sense and not in a haphazard sense. This is achieved by using a random number generator to sample elements from the population. Suppose we wish to have a sample of 100 from our population of 3,191 counties and county equivalents. There are two approaches to simple random sampling—with replacement and without replacement to get a sample of 100 counties.

With replacement, the first county has a 1 in 3,191 chance of selection. Once the county is selected, we do not remove the county from our listing. Because the county selected is not removed from the list (essentially, "replaced" in the list), the chance of selection of the second to 100th sample is also 1 in 3,191.

Under simple random sampling without replacement, the first county has a 1 in 3,191 chance of selection. Because the selected county is not replaced in our listing, the second county to be selected has a 1 in 3,190 (since the first selected county has been removed from the list) chance of selection. Now for the third county to be selected, the chance of selection is 1 in 3,189 (since two counties have been selected and removed from the list). For each subsequent selection, the list of counties available for selection keeps reducing as the selected counties are not replaced.

10.3.1.1 RANDOM NUMBER GENERATION IN EXCEL

In our example in Excel, we use the random number generator to make our selection, with or without replacement. Open Dataset 19 and label the cell G1 "Random Number" and the cell H1 "Random Number Fixed" (Figure 10.2). Next, in cell G2, type the formula "=RAND( )"—this is the formula for generating a random number—and press "Enter." You will notice that the number "0" appears in the cell. This is because the cell has not been formatted for numbers with decimal values. Go ahead and select the entire columns

---

Tutorial video for Section 10.3.1 is available by accessing the following url: https://connect .springerpub.com/content/book/978-0-8261-5028-8/chapter/ch11

STATE COI	COUNTY C State	County	Percent of population that is female	Percent of Population living in a rural area	Random Number	Random Number Fixed
1	0 AL	Alabama	0.515	0.41	=RAND()	
1	1 AL	Autauga County	0.514	0.42		
1	3 AL	Baldwin County	0.512	0.423		
1	5 AL	Barbour County	0.466	0.678		
1	7 AL	Bibb County	0.459	0.684		
1	9 AL	Blount County	0.505	0.9		
1	11 AL	Bullock County	0.453	0.514		
1	13 AL	Butler County	0.536	0.712		
1	15 AL	Calhoun County	0.518	0.337		
1	17 AL	Chambers County	0.523	0.491		
1	19 AL	Cherokee County	0.502	0.857		
1	21 AL	Chilton County	0.508	0.867		
1	23 AL	Choctaw County	0.525	1		
1	25 AL	Clarke County	0.528	0.76		
1	27 AL	Clay County	0.506	1		
1	29 AL	Cleburne County	0.504	1		
1	31 AL	Coffee County	0.505	0.472		
1	33 AL	Colbert County	0.518	0.439		
1	35 AL	Conecuh County	0.519	0.809		
1	37 AL	Coosa County	0.495	1		
1	39 AL	Covington County	0.516	0.697		
1	41 AL	Crenshaw County	0.511	1		
1	43 AL	Cullman County	0.505	0.732		
1	45 AL	Dale County	0.505	0.509		
1	47 AL	Dallas County	0.537	0.456		
1	49 AL	DeKalb County	0.507	0.901		
1	51 AL	Elmore County	0.515	0.542		
1	53 AL	Escambia County	0.498	0.635		

2016 Listing of Counties in the

FIGURE 10.2 Random number for simple random sampling.

G and H (click on "G"; hold down the "shift" key and click on "H") and right click to choose "Format Cell" and click the tab for "Number." Here, under "Category" choose "Number" and make sure to have four decimal places. Now, go back to cell G2 and click in the cell such that the cell is bordered and there is a small square on the bottom right of the border. Hold down this square and drag and copy it down the entire column to the last row with data in this list—row 3,192.

The random numbers that we have just generated are dynamic. Because they are based on the computer's clock, these random numbers are not fixed and will constantly keep changing. For this reason, we have created the column "Random Number Fixed" in order to paste the values there. To do this, we first click on the last cell (G3192) with the random number, hold down the "control" and "shift" keys and press the "up-arrow" key. Once all the cells with random numbers and the column title are highlighted, release all keys and hold down the S"shift" key and click on cell G2 (just below the column header). On the "Home" ribbon, choose "Copy." Next, click on cell H2 and on "Home" ribbon, click the "down arrow" under "Paste" and select "Paste Values" (Figure 10.3). As you paste the values, you will notice that all the random numbers in the column "Random number" change. Now that you have pasted the values of these random numbers in column H, these values will not constantly change.

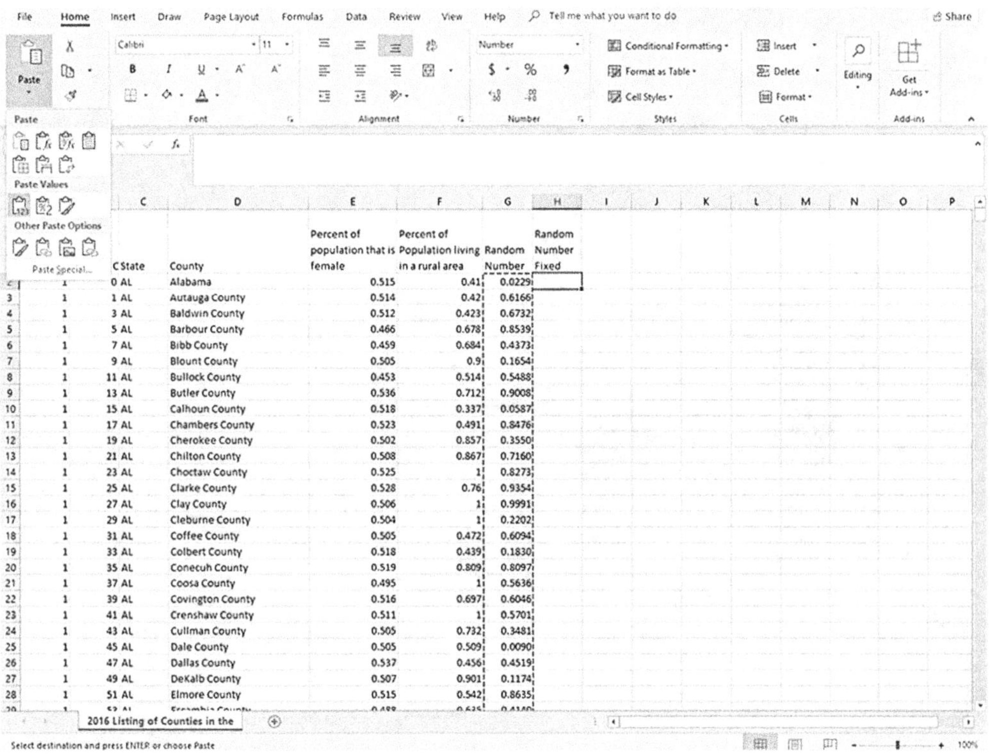

C State	County	Percent of population that is female	Percent of Population living in a rural area	Random Number	Random Number Fixed
0 AL	Alabama	0.515	0.41	0.0229	
1 AL	Autauga County	0.514	0.42	0.6166	
3 AL	Baldwin County	0.512	0.423	0.6732	
5 AL	Barbour County	0.466	0.678	0.8539	
7 AL	Bibb County	0.459	0.684	0.4373	
9 AL	Blount County	0.505	0.9	0.1654	
11 AL	Bullock County	0.453	0.514	0.5488	
13 AL	Butler County	0.536	0.712	0.9008	
15 AL	Calhoun County	0.518	0.337	0.0587	
17 AL	Chambers County	0.523	0.491	0.8476	
19 AL	Cherokee County	0.502	0.857	0.3550	
21 AL	Chilton County	0.508	0.867	0.7160	
23 AL	Choctaw County	0.525	1	0.8273	
25 AL	Clarke County	0.528	0.76	0.9354	
27 AL	Clay County	0.506	1	0.9991	
29 AL	Cleburne County	0.504	1	0.2202	
31 AL	Coffee County	0.505	0.472	0.6094	
33 AL	Colbert County	0.518	0.439	0.1830	
35 AL	Conecuh County	0.519	0.809	0.8097	
37 AL	Coosa County	0.495	1	0.5636	
39 AL	Covington County	0.516	0.697	0.6046	
41 AL	Crenshaw County	0.511	1	0.5701	
43 AL	Cullman County	0.505	0.732	0.3481	
45 AL	Dale County	0.505	0.509	0.0090	
47 AL	Dallas County	0.537	0.456	0.4519	
49 AL	DeKalb County	0.507	0.901	0.1174	
51 AL	Elmore County	0.515	0.542	0.8635	
53 AL	Escambia County	0.488	0.635	0.4140	

2016 Listing of Counties in the

FIGURE 10.3 Copying and pasting random number values.

Now to choose our first county, we can go ahead and sort the column containing the fixed random numbers and pick the county with the lowest value. To do this, click on cell A1 and hold down the "control" and "shift" keys and press the "right arrow" and then press the "down arrow." Click on "Data" in the toolbar and then select "Sort" from the "Sort and Filter" group in the ribbon (Figure 10.4). In the "Sort" panel, make sure to choose "Random Number Fixed" as the column to "Sort by," check the box for "My data has headers," and select "Smallest to Largest" under "Order."

In our example, Knox county in Ohio comes up as the county with the smallest fixed random number. If we were doing simple random sampling with replacement, we would copy Knox county in our sample list and then resort the list of all counties by "State Code" and "County Code." Once the counties are resorted back to the original, we will start by copying the random numbers from column G and pasting the values in column H (as described earlier in this section), and then sorting the "Random Number Fixed" to make our next selection, and so on.

For simple random sampling without replacement, the procedure is the same as "with replacement," except that each time we will remove the county selected in our sample and proceed with the resorting, random number generation, and fixing value before sorting.

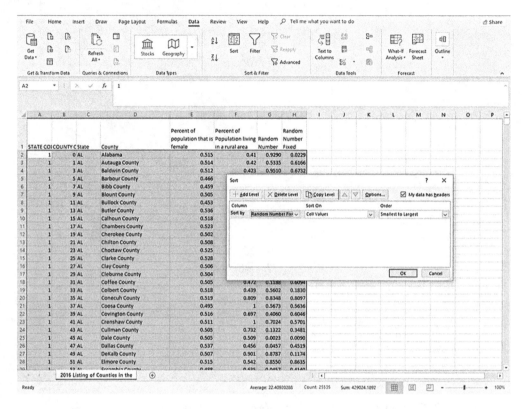

FIGURE 10.4 Sorting random number values.

10.3.2 Systematic Random Sampling

This is a variant of simple random sampling. As in simple random sampling, the first sample selection is done through the random number generator and sorting as described previously. Once this first sample is selected, the remaining elements in the sample are simply identified by choosing the appropriate sampling interval (i) and choosing every ith element in our list to get all elements in the sample. In our example with 3,191 counties and county equivalents, after identifying the first sample randomly, the sorted list of the remaining 3,190 counties and county equivalents would be divided by the remaining sample size required (99) to get the sampling interval (3,190/99 ~ 32). Thus, every 32nd element in our list would then be chosen to get our sample size of 100.

10.3.3 Stratified Random Sampling

Stratified random sampling is used when we have data on a variable of interest that could be used to stratify or create layers for sampling. For instance,

---

Tutorial video for Section 10.3.2 is available by accessing the following url: https://connect .springerpub.com/content/book/978-0-8261-5028-8/chapter/ch11

Tutorial video for Section 10.3.3 is available by accessing the following url: https://connect .springerpub.com/content/book/978-0-8261-5028-8/chapter/ch11

if we were undertaking a study where our variable of interest is rural areas. In this study, we can use the known percentage of rural counties in the U.S. to stratify rural and urban areas. If the known percentage of rural counties in the U.S. is hypothetically 60%. Under this approach, being interested in generating a random sample of 100 counties from our list of 3,191, we could resort to two variants to get our sample:

a. Proportionate stratified sampling—Here, instead of selecting 100 counties for this study through a random sampling of the list of all counties in the U.S., we change our approach. We split the list of counties into two—list of rural counties and list of urban counties. Then, from the list of rural counties, we use random sampling to select 60 rural counties and from the list of urban counties we use random sampling to select 40 urban counties. Now our stratified sample of 100 counties has 60 rural counties and 40 urban counties. Thus the proportion of rural counties in our sample is 60/100 = 60%.

b. Disproportionate stratified sampling—Under this approach, we use our lists of urban and rural counties to randomly sample counties. However, instead of the number of urban and rural counties being proportionate to the percent of rural counties in the United States, we might sample 50 counties from rural and 50 counties from the urban list.

10.3.4 Cluster Sampling

In order to balance the needs of drawing a random sample and the real costs of having our sample of counties literally all over the map and the exorbitant costs of data collection in all these places, sometimes cluster sampling is used. Under this approach, the random sampling happens in two or more stages. As before, if we are interested in generating a random sample of 100 counties from our list of 3,191, we would use stages to make the data collection more manageable. For instance, our first stage could be to identify through random sampling 10 states and within these 10 states to identify counties such that we have a sample of 100 counties. Here, the first stage of selecting states could be based on the simple random or systematic random sampling. Once the 10 states are thus identified, then the process of random sampling is applied to the next stage (list of counties in the 10 selected states) to get our sample of 100 counties. This selection at the second stage of the number of counties per state can be equal for each state (i.e., 10 per state) or it can be proportionate

Tutorial video for Section 10.3.4 is available by accessing the following url: https://connect .springerpub.com/content/book/978-0-8261-5028-8/chapter/ch11

to the size of the population or the number of representatives in the House of Representatives from the state.

10.4 Nonprobability Sampling

We now consider nonprobability sampling approaches. Unlike probability sampling, here the chance or probability of an element from the population being selected is not known in advance of the study. These approaches are frequently used for qualitative-focused studies. In order to illustrate the differences between probabilistic and nonprobabilistic sampling, we will continue to use our example of 100 county samples.

There are four broad approaches to nonprobability sampling—availability (convenience), quota, purposive, and snowball.

10.4.1 Availability (Convenience) Sampling

As the name suggests, this is just choosing samples that are conveniently available. For instance, if you need to interview 30 people for a study, you ask your coworkers to be study respondents. In our example of selecting 100 counties, availability or convenience sampling would be choosing the 100 counties closest to where you reside.

10.4.2 Quota Sampling

Under quota sampling, the sample size is divided to ensure that certain characteristics of the population are there in the sample. For instance, in your 30-people study, if you are interested in your sample representing racial characteristics at your workplace, you would establish quotas or numbers for each race to ensure that your sample has the same racial characteristics. In your example of 100 counties study, if there are 60% rural counties in the United States, you would have a quota of 60 of the 100 counties in your sample being rural. Unlike stratified random sampling where we also have a sample that includes 60 rural counties, here, under quota sampling, the 60 rural counties would not be chosen randomly or probabilistically.

10.4.3 Purposive Sampling

For purposive sampling, the entire sample is selected because of certain unique characteristics. For instance, in your 30-person study, if you are interested in studying long-distance commuting, you would choose your sample from among long-distance commuters at your workplace. In your 100-county study, if you are studying the effect of low health insurance rates, you would purposively choose counties where the health insurance rate is low.

10.4.4 Snowball Sampling

A rolling snowball collects more snow as it rolls along. In the same way, the sample here builds up based on suggestions from people you interview as to whom else you could interview. In the 30-person study about long-distance commute, you may start with one person you know who commutes long distance. After interviewing that person, you would ask whom else he or she knows who commutes long distance and could be interviewed for this study. The process would continue with each successive interviewee providing additional names of persons you could interview.

10.5 Research Design

The purpose for research has implications for research design. Broadly, research is undertaken for three main reasons—explore, describe, or test a phenomenon, concept, or relationship (Singleton & Straits, 2010). Of these three reasons, exploratory studies are less structured because we are studying something that we do not understand completely, and flexibility is built into the research process. However, for studies that either seek to describe or test a phenomenon, concept, or relationship, the research design is structured.

Research design includes three key elements (Schutt, 2015)—unit of analysis, cross-sectional or longitudinal data, and methods (qualitative/ quantitative/mixed).

10.5.1 Unit of Analysis

Data collection can be undertaken at various levels—individual, family, group, city, state, country, and so on. However, much of primary data collection occurs at the individual level. Depending on the research question, the unit of analysis may not be the same as the unit of data collection. In case of a mismatch between the unit of data collection and unit of analysis, errors in inference may occur as under the following (Schutt, 2015; Singleton & Straits, 2010):

a. Reductionist or individual fallacy: If data collected at the individual level are analyzed to make inferences about the group.

b. Ecological fallacy: If group-level data are analyzed to make inferences about individuals.

10.5.2 Cross-Sectional or Longitudinal Data

As part of the research design, the collection of data could be at one time (cross-sectional) or at two or more times (longitudinal). When data collection is across two or more time periods, there are some differences as to whether the data are collected from the same individuals (fixed panel) or if it collected from different individuals (repeated cross-sectional).

10.5.3 Methods

The third element of research design covers the methods used for the research. Depending on the research question and the explanation guiding the study, researchers may choose from the following:

a. Quantitative methods: Here, variations in the independent variable are followed by variations in the dependent variable, when everything else is held constant.

b. Qualitative methods: These methods are used when specific events and actions are thought to result in particular outcomes.

c. Mixed methods: As the name suggests, this is a hybrid of quantitative and qualitative methods and would have a focus on one of the methods while including the other method. By including a hybrid approach, the intent is to use a much broader approach to explaining the phenomenon being studied.

A "whimsical" way to understand how these three methods come together and have a role to play is very succinctly portrayed in the AHRQ report (Johnson et al., 2015). Figure 10.5 describes the flow (pun intended) of the

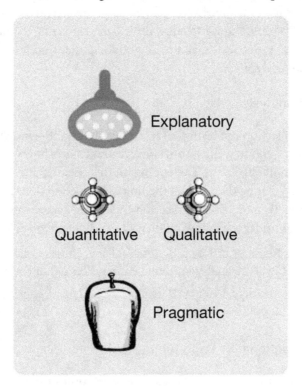

FIGURE 10.5 Flow of analytical methods.
SOURCE: Johnson, K., Gustafson, D., Ewigman, B., Provost, L., & Roper, R. (2015). *Using rapid-cycle research to reach goals: Awareness, assessment, adaptation, acceleration* (AHRQ Publication No. 15-0036). Rockville, MD: Agency for Healthcare Research and Quality. Retrieved from https://pbrn.ahrq.gov/sites/default/files/docs/page/AHRQPBRNFinalRapidCycleResearchGuidanceDocument_1.pdf

different methods and the attendant resources. Based on the research question or problem that ranges from explanatory to the pragmatic, one can choose a combination of quantitative, qualitative, or mixed approaches—the faucets in Figure 10.5. Depending on which faucets are chosen and how much they are turned on, the resources may be a trickle (showerhead) or come gushing out to fill the tub.

This brief overview of the process of sampling and research design is to provide an appreciation of some of the issues involved and their implications for analysis and hypothesis testing.

10.6 Competency Development

In Box 10.1, we are introduced to the AHRQ's approach to RCR. Here, AHRQ is putting forth the steps that will help research design to evolve to keep pace with changes in healthcare delivery such as horizontal and vertical integration. This is to hasten the pace of research to actionable insights that will address quality improvement as well as implementation of interventions. In this approach, the working definition of RCR emphasizes the need to start with identifying practical problems and ensuring that analytical methods are based on the context where these problems occur. The six phases of RCR range from identification of stakeholders all the way to implementation and dissemination. Through this phased approach to actionable research, there is clear application of skills from the competency domain of critical thinking.

Next, practical aspects of analysis and hypothesis testing require appreciation of the process of sampling to understand sample estimates and population values. This appreciation also helps with the generalizability of results. Thus, common approaches to probabilistic and nonprobabilistic sampling are explored, including how Excel can be used for random sampling. These steps ensure application of skills from the competency domain of problem-solving.

For all research and analysis, the starting point is always a well-identified research question. This research question has implications for research design. Other than for exploratory research, the research design is structured—even for RCR. The research design includes considerations related to unit of analysis, cross-sectional or longitudinal data, and quantitative, qualitative, or mixed methods. In relating our research question to research design, we engage in application of skills from the competency domain of critical thinking.

By appreciating the need for research to evolve to the ever-changing healthcare environment and using problems and questions as the basis for research, we focus on the competency domain of critical thinking. Next, by understanding research design and applying sampling using Excel, we focus on the competency domains of critical thinking and problem-solving.

10.7 Summary

There are rapid changes in the healthcare environment on account of vertical and horizontal integration that are precipitating the need for research to evolve to address quality improvement and interventions. The RCR framework underscores the need to start with a problem and then use a systematic approach to research to address the problem. In order to best use research, a broad understanding of the more common methods of probability and nonprobability sampling and application of these methods through Excel are important. There are several research design considerations that are suited to the question that we are trying to answer. Lastly, quantitative, qualitative, and mixed methods are available for use within our chosen research designs.

10.8 Discussion Questions

10.8.1 Identify specific changes in the healthcare environment. How are these changes driving the need for research to evolve?

10.8.2 Suppose you are overseeing a public health department and are concerned about one county as having poor health outcomes. What would you do to address this problem?

10.8.3 How are random and nonrandom sampling approaches different and similar?

10.8.4 What is the most important element of research design? Why?

10.9 Practice Problems

(▶)   All datasets required for the practice problems are available for download at http://connect.springerpub.com/content/book/978-0-8261-5028-8.

10.9.1 You are working with the executive team at the Veterans Administration (VA). Your team would like to focus the attention of the executive team on specific issues that are flagged in the Consumer Assessment of Healthcare Providers and Systems in VA facilities. Rather than show data from all facilities, you consider using simple random sampling to select 30 VA facilities from Dataset 3. Use this file to identify two different simple random samples:

a. Simple random sampling with replacement

b. Simple random sampling without replacement

c. For each of the abtwo samples, provide the average value for the variable "Recommend Hospital."

(▶) Tutorial videos provided for Practice Problems 10.9.1—10.9.7 can be accessed by accessing the following url: https://connect.springerpub.com/content/book/978-0-8261-5028-8/chapter/ch11

10.9.2 You are working with the executive team at the Veterans Administration (VA). Your team would like to focus the attention of the executive team on specific issues that are flagged in the Consumer Assessment of Healthcare Providers and Systems in VA facilities. Rather than show data from all facilities, you consider using systematic random sampling to select 30 VA facilities from Dataset 3. Use this file to identify your sample of 30 facilities.

a. For your sample, provide the average value for the variable "Recommend Hospital."

10.9.3 You are working with the executive team at the Veterans Administration (VA). Your team would like to focus the attention of the executive team on specific issues that are flagged in the Consumer Assessment of Healthcare Providers and Systems in VA facilities. Rather than show data from all facilities, you consider using stratified random sampling to select 40 VA facilities from Dataset 3. Use quartiles of the variable "Recommend Hospital" to create four strata and then identify 10 facilities from each stratum.

a. For your sample, provide the average value for the variable "Recommend Hospital."

10.9.4 You are working with the executive team at the Veterans Administration (VA). Your team would like to focus the attention of the executive team on specific issues that are flagged in the Consumer Assessment of Healthcare Providers and Systems in VA facilities. Rather than show data from all facilities, you consider using convenience sampling to select 30 VA facilities from Dataset 3. Use this file to identify your sample of 30 facilities.

a. For your sample, provide the average value for the variable "Recommend Hospital."

10.9.5 You are working with the executive team at the Veterans Administration (VA). Your team would like to focus the attention of the executive team on specific issues that are flagged in the Consumer Assessment of Healthcare Providers and Systems in VA facilities. Rather than show data from all facilities, you consider using purposive sampling to select 30 VA facilities from Dataset 3. Use the variable "Recommend Hospital" to identify your sample of 30 facilities.

a. For your sample, provide the average value for the variable "Recommend Hospital."

10.9.6 You are in the national office of the Centers for Medicare and Medicaid Services (CMS). For a study on how Medicare recipients may be sampled to answer brief questions on different approaches to Medicare for All, how would you go about designing a representative study? Consider design as well as sampling issues and use Dataset 19 to provide a sampling of counties that you would include in your study.

10.9.7 You are in the national office of the CMS. For a state-level study on Medicaid expansion, how would you go about designing a representative study? Consider design as well as sampling issues and use Dataset 9 to provide a sampling of states that you would include in your study.

See Chapter 11, Video Tutorials and Answers to Practice Problems Using Healthcare Datasets in Excel®, for video answers to the practice problems.

References

Johnson, K., Gustafson, D., Ewigman, B., Provost, L., & Roper, R. (2015). *Using rapid-cycle research to reach goals: Awareness, assessment, adaptation, acceleration* Rockville, MD: Agency for Healthcare Research and Quality. https://pbrn.ahrq .gov/sites/default/files/docs/page/AHRQPBRNFinalRapidCycleResearch GuidanceDocument_1.pdf

Schutt, R. K. (2015). *Investigating the social world: The process and practice of research* (8th ed.). Thousand Oaks, CA: Sage.

Singleton, R., Jr., & Straits, B. C. (2010). *Approaches to social research* (5th ed.). New York, NY: Oxford University Press.

VIDEO TUTORIALS AND ANSWERS TO PRACTICE PROBLEMS USING HEALTHCARE DATASETS IN EXCEL®

This textbook uses a competency-based approach to promote application of the use of Excel® for analysis of healthcare data. What better way to promote this application than to supplement the use in each chapter of screen capture with videos that provide the step-by-step interface between Excel and healthcare data for these applications. The use of step-by-step video tutorials takes the next step in ensuring that there are no gaps in understanding how the capabilities of Excel are used with healthcare data. At the same time, this more comprehensive video-based approach will also appeal to learners who may learn better through a video demonstration rather than a more restricted text-based approach with screen captures, as well as online learners who may not have the benefit of in-class instructions on these applications. These video tutorials are not limited just to the screen captures of application of Excel to healthcare data. They also extend to video solutions for all end-of-chapter practice problems.

Please use the url (or QR code) provided at the bottom of the page to access video tutorials, on the screen captures, as well as solutions to practice problems. All videos are in MP4 format.

Chapter 2: Working in Excel® and Importing Healthcare Data

 2.4.1–2.4.2 Importing Data and Managing Worksheets

2.5.1 to 2.5.2 Aligning Content and Visual Examination

2.6.1 Highlighting and Counting Blank Cells

2.6.2 Swapping Rows and Columns

2.6.4 Splitting Fields

2.6.5 Combining Fields

2.7 Managing Add-Ins in Excel

 Tutorial videos: https://connect.springerpub.com/content/book/978-0-8261-5028-8/chapter/ch11

Chapter 7: Visualization and Spatial Analysis of Healthcare Data Using 3D Maps in Excel®

Chapter 8: Using Analysis of Variance (ANOVA) in Healthcare Datasets to Compare Groups and Test Hypotheses in Excel®

LIST OF SELECT SOURCES OF HEALTHCARE DATA

DATA	CATEGORY	DESCRIPTION	WEBSITE
American Community Survey (ACS)	Population survey	ACS is conducted by the U.S. Census Bureau and provides social, housing, and economic characteristics for demographic groups covering a broad spectrum of geographic areas in the United States and Puerto Rico.	https://www.census .gov/programs -surveys/acs/data .html
American Housing Survey (AHS)	Population survey	AHS is conducted by the U.S. Census Bureau and provides information on a national sample of housing units, including single-family homes, apartments, mobile homes, and vacant homes.	https://www.census .gov/programs -surveys/ahs/data .html
American Time Use Survey (ATUS)	Population survey	ATUS is conducted by the U.S. Dept. of Labor: Bureau of Labor Statistics and collects information on how U.S. adults spent their time during the past day on activities such as paid work, childcare, volunteering, religious activities, etc.	https://www.bls.gov/ tus/#data

(continued)

This select list of sources of healthcare data has been developed through the Digital Humanities Seed Grant from the Center for Faculty Development, Seton Hall University, 2018–19, that was awarded to the author.

DATA	CATEGORY	DESCRIPTION	WEBSITE
Annual Survey of Governments: Financial Statistics	Administrative records	This annual survey is conducted by the U.S. Census to provide periodic and comprehensive statistics about governments and governmental financial activities such as revenue and expenditure as well as by accounting categories.	https://www.census .gov/programs- surveys/state/data/ tables.All.html
CBS News Blitz Poll	Population survey	This poll conducted by CBS/*New York Times* asked respondents their opinion about VA medical facilities.	https://www.icpsr .umich.edu/icpsrweb/ ICPSR/studies/ 36199/version/1/ datadocumentation
Census of Public and Private Juvenile Detention Correctional and Shelter Facilities	Administrative records	This census is conducted by the U.S. Dept. of Justice and provides information on the population and characteristics of public and private juvenile facilities in the United States.	https://www.icpsr .umich.edu/icpsrweb/ NACJD/studies/ 24260/version/2/ datadocumentation
Census of State and Federal Adult Correctional Facilities	Administrative records	This census is conducted by the U.S. Bureau of Census on behalf of the Dept. of Justice and contains information on inmates and incidents, including deaths at adult correctional facilities in the United States.	https://www.icpsr .umich.edu/icpsrweb/ NACJD/studies/ 24642/version/3/ datadocumentation
Child Care Licensing Study	Administrative records	This study conducted by the Department of Health and Human Services and the National Association of Regulatory Administration provides information about childcare licensing programs and policies and the regulations for childcare centers in all 50 states, D.C., and territories of the United States.	https://www .researchconnections .org/childcare/ studies/37026/ versions/V1/ datadocumentation
Community Tracking Study: Household Survey	Population survey	Conducted by the Center for Studying Health System Change and sponsored by the Robert Wood Johnson Foundation, this national study tracks changes in the U.S. healthcare system and its effects using a sample of households.	https://www.icpsr .umich.edu/icpsrweb/ HMCA/studies/ 04216/version/2/ datadocumentation

(continued)

DATA	CATEGORY	DESCRIPTION	WEBSITE
Community Tracking Study: Physician Survey	Provider survey	Conducted by the Center for Studying Health System Change and sponsored by the Robert Wood Johnson Foundation, this national study tracks changes in the U.S. healthcare system and its effects using a sample of physicians.	https://www.icpsr .umich.edu/icpsrweb/ HMCA/studies/ 04584/version/2/ datadocumentation
County Health Rankings—Links to State Data	Population survey	A variety of state-specific health and social services data with links provided through the County Health Rankings and Roadmaps.	http://www .countyhealthrankings .org/explore-health -rankings/use-the -data/go-beyond -the-snapshot/ find-more-data
Criminal Justice Drug Abuse Treatment Studies: Organizational Process Improvement Interventions	Provider survey	This study is maintained by the National Addiction and HIV Data Archive Program and provides access to imple- mentation research in criminal justice settings.	https://www.icpsr .umich.edu/icpsrweb/ NAHDAP/data/ index.jsp
Current Population Survey: Tobacco Use Supplement	Population survey	This monthly survey is con- ducted by the U.S. Dept. of Labor and includes a tobacco use supplement.	https://www.icpsr .umich.edu/icpsrweb/ ICPSR/studies/36845/ version/1/ datadocumentation
Deaths in Custody Reporting Program: Jail Populations	Administrative records	This study is conducted by the U.S. Dept. of Justice and collects data on inmates dying in state prisons.	https://www.icpsr .umich.edu/icpsrweb/ NACJD/studies/ 36560/version/1/ datadocumentation
Family Interaction, Social Capital, and Trends in Time Use	Population survey	This study conducted by the University of Maryland col- lected information on social capital and life quality.	https://www.icpsr .umich.edu/icpsrweb/ ICPSR/studies/03191/ version/1/ datadocumentation
General Social Survey	Population survey	This study is conducted by the National Opinion Research Center at the University of Chicago and provides a time- lapse study of changes in societal trends, attitudes, and behaviors.	http://gss.norc.org/ Get-The-Data

(continued)

DATA	CATEGORY	DESCRIPTION	WEBSITE
Health Behavior in School-Age Children	Population survey	This study is conducted by the U.S. Dept. of Health and Human Services and sponsored by the World Health Organization.	https://www.uib.no/en/hbscdata
Health Information National Trends Survey (HINTS)	Population survey	HINTS is conducted by the National Institutes of Health: National Cancer Institute and is a nationally representative study about people's access to and use of cancer-related information.	https://hints.cancer.gov
Health Reform Monitoring Survey	Population survey	This survey is conducted by the Urban Institute among the nonelderly population to explore the use of cutting-edge Internet-based survey methods on a variety of topics on healthcare reform.	https://www.icpsr.umich.edu/icpsrweb/HMCA/studies/36744/version/1/datadocumentation
Health Tracking Household Survey	Population survey	This survey is conducted by the Center for Studying Health System Change and is the successor to the Community Tracking Survey and this national study tracks changes in the U.S. healthcare system and its effects using a sample of households.	https://www.icpsr.umich.edu/icpsrweb/HMCA/studies/34141/version/1/datadocumentation
Health Tracking Physician Survey	Provider survey	This survey is conducted by the Center for Studying Health System Change and is the successor to the Community Tracking Survey and this national study tracks changes in the U.S. healthcare system and its effects using a sample of physicians.	https://www.icpsr.umich.edu/icpsrweb/HMCA/studies/27202/version/1/datadocumentation
Hispanic Established Populations for the Epidemiologic Study of the Elderly	Population survey	This survey is maintained by the National Archive of Computerized Data on Aging (NACDA) and provides data on risk factors for mortality and morbidity in Mexican Americans in order to contrast how these factors operate differently in non-Hispanic White Americans, African Americans, and other major ethnic groups.	https://www.icpsr.umich.edu/icpsrweb/NACDA/studies/36578/version/2/datadocumentation

(continued)

DATA	CATEGORY	DESCRIPTION	WEBSITE
Hospital Consumer Assessment of Healthcare Providers and Systems (HCAHPS)	Population survey	This survey is published by the Centers for Medicare and Medicaid Services and collects information from patients and their experiences at hospitals.	https://catalog.data .gov/dataset/patient -survey-hcahps -hospital
Linked Birth/ Infant Death Period Data	Vital statistics	As part of the National Vital Statistics System, the linked birth and infant death dataset is a valuable tool that connects information from the death certificate to information from the birth certificate for each infant under 1 year of age who dies in the United States, Puerto Rico, The Virgin Islands, and Guam.	https://www .cdc.gov/nchs/nvss/ linked-birth .htm#Two_Formats
Medicare Current Beneficiary Survey: Access to Care	Population survey	This survey is conducted by the Centers for Medicare and Medicaid Services and is a representative sample of the elderly and disabled beneficiaries and their access to medical care.	https://www.cms.gov/ Research-Statistics -Data-and-Systems/ Research/MCBS/ Data-Tables.html
Mortality Detail File	Vital statistics	Available through the Centers for Disease Control and Prevention: National Center for Health Statistics, it provides details on every registered death in the United States.	https://www.cdc.gov/ nchs/data_access/ VitalStatsOnline.htm
Multiple Cause of Death Public Use Files	Registry of diseases	Available through the Centers for Disease Control and Prevention (CDC), the Multiple Cause of Death database contains mortality and population counts for all U.S. counties.	https://wonder.cdc .gov/mcd-icd10.html
Natality Detail File	Vital statistics	Available through the Centers for Disease Control and Prevention: National Center for Health Statistics, it provides details on every live birth in the United States.	https://www.cdc .gov/nchs/nvss/birth_ methods.htm

(continued)

DATA	CATEGORY	DESCRIPTION	WEBSITE
National Ambulatory Medical Care Survey	Provider survey	Available through the Centers for Disease Control and Prevention: National Center for Health Statistics, it provides details on a sample of visits to non-federally funded ambulatory medical care settings in the United States.	https://www.cdc.gov/nchs/ahcd/datasets_documentation_related.htm
National Comorbidity Survey: Reinterview	Population survey	The study is maintained by the National Addiction and HIV Data Archive Program and was conducted a decade after the initial baseline survey and provides information about changes in mental disorders, substance use disorders, and the predictors and consequences of these changes over the 10 years between the two surveys.	https://www.icpsr.umich.edu/icpsrweb/NAHDAP/studies/35067/version/2/datadocumentation
National Electronic Injury Surveillance System	Provider survey	This study is conducted by the Centers for Disease Control and Prevention: National Center for Injury Prevention and Control and the Consumer Product Safety Commission, and collects data on injuries in a nationally representative sample of hospitals with emergency departments.	https://www.cpsc.gov/Research--Statistics/NEISS-Injury-Data
National Health and Nutrition Examination Survey	Population survey	This survey is conducted by the Centers for Disease Control and Prevention: National Center for Health Statistics and collects information on health and nutritional status of adults and children through interviews and physical examination.	https://wwwn.cdc.gov/nchs/nhanes/Default.aspx
National Health Expenditure	Administrative records	These data are maintained through the Centers for Medicare and Medicaid Services on the sources of funds and types of health expenditure at the national level.	https://www.cms.gov/Research-Statistics-Data-and-Systems/Statistics-Trends-and-Reports/NationalHealthExpendData/NationalHealthAccountsHistorical.html

(continued)

DATA	CATEGORY	DESCRIPTION	WEBSITE
National Home and Hospice Care Survey	Provider survey	This survey, last conducted in 2007 by the Centers for Disease Control and Prevention: National Center for Health Statistics, collects information on home health and hospice agencies, their staffs, their services, and their patients.	https://www.icpsr .umich.edu/icpsrweb/ NACDA/studies/ 28961/version/1/ datadocumentation
National Hospital Ambulatory Medical Care Survey	Provider survey	This survey is conducted by the Centers for Disease Control and Prevention: National Center for Health Statistics and collects information on a national sample of hospitals and patients in their outpatient and emergency departments.	https://www.cdc.gov/ nchs/ahcd/datasets_ documentation_ related.htm
National Hospital Discharge Survey	Provider survey	This survey, conducted from 1965 to 2010 by the Centers for Disease Control and Prevention: National Center for Health Statistics, collects information on a sample of nonfederal short-stay hospitals and inpatients discharged from these hospitals.	https://www.cdc.gov/ nchs/nhds/nhds_ questionnaires.htm
National Immunization Survey	Population survey	This is a phone-based survey conducted by the National Opinion Research Center, University of Chicago, under the directions of the Centers for Disease Control and Prevention: National Center for Immunization and Respiratory Diseases and collects information on vaccination coverage among children and teens, including flu vaccination.	https://www.cdc.gov/ nchs/nis/data_ files.htm
National Institute for Child Health and Human Development (NICHD) Study of Early Child Care and Youth Development	Population survey	This study, conducted by the National Institutes of Health: National Institute for Child Health and Human Development, examines the influence of variations in early childcare histories on the psychological development of infants and toddlers from a variety of family backgrounds.	https://www.icpsr .umich.edu/icpsrweb/ DSDR/studies/22361/ versions/V5/ datadocumentation

(continued)

DATA	CATEGORY	DESCRIPTION	WEBSITE
National Mental Health Services Survey	Population survey	This survey is conducted by the Department of Health and Human Services: Substance Abuse and Mental Health Services Administration and collects information from all mental health treatment facilities in the United States, including patient information every other year.	https://www .datafiles.samhsa .gov/study-series/ national-mental- health-services- survey-n-mhss- nid13521
National Mortality Followback Survey	Population survey	This survey is conducted by the Centers for Disease Control and Prevention: National Center for Health Statistics and samples U.S. residents 15 years and older who died and provides information from their death certificates and other sources.	https://www.cdc.gov /nchs/nvss/nmfs/ nmfs_methods.htm
National Nursing Home Survey	Provider survey	This survey, conducted till 2004 by the Centers for Disease Control and Prevention: National Center for Health Statistics, collects information on a nationally representative sample of nursing homes, their staffs, their residents, and services.	https://www.cdc.gov/ nchs/nnhs/nnhs_ questionnaires.htm
National Social Life, Health and Aging Project	Population survey	This survey is conducted by the National Opinion Research Center, University of Chicago, among a national sample of older community-dwelling Americans on a host of social, demographic, and health factors.	https://www.icpsr .umich.edu/icpsrweb/ NACDA/studies/ 36873/versions/V4/ datadocumentation
National Study of Long-Term Care Providers		This biennial survey is conducted by the Centers for Disease Control and Prevention: National Center for Health Statistics and provides data on residential and adult day care, home health, nursing home, and hospice care.	https://www.cdc.gov/ nchs/nsltcp/nsltcp_ questionnaires.htm

(continued)

DATA	CATEGORY	DESCRIPTION	WEBSITE
National Survey of Alcohol, Drug, and Mental Health Problems	Population survey	This survey is part of the Robert Wood Johnson–funded Health Tracking Initiative.	https://www.icpsr.umich.edu/icpsrweb/HMCA/studies/04165/version/1/datadocumentation
National Survey of America's Families	Population survey	This is a household survey conducted by the Urban Institute to collect data on the well-being of children, adults, and families.	https://www.researchconnections.org/childcare/studies/04582/version/1/datadocumentation
National Survey of Black Americans	Population survey	This is a study conducted by the University of Michigan: Institute for Social Research to collect data on neighborhood, societal, demographic, religious, cultural, and economic factors in the lives of Black Americans.	https://www.icpsr.umich.edu/icpsrweb/NACDA/studies/06668/version/1/datadocumentation
National Survey of Children's Exposure to Violence	Population survey	This study, conducted by the University of New Hampshire, collects data on lifetime and 1-year incidence estimates of a range of childhood victimization incidents.	https://www.icpsr.umich.edu/icpsrweb/NACJD/studies/35203/version/1/datadocumentation
National Survey of Children's Health	Population survey	This survey is conducted by the Centers for Disease Control and Prevention: National Center for Health Statistics to produce national and state estimates on a range of indicators related to children's interaction with the healthcare system.	https://www.census.gov/programs-surveys/nsch/data/data-tool.html
National Survey of Family Growth	Population survey	This survey is conducted by the Centers for Disease Control and Prevention: National Center for Health Statistics and collects data on family life, marriage and divorce, pregnancy, infertility, use of contraception, and men's and women's health.	https://www.cdc.gov/nchs/nsfg/nsfg_questionnaires.htm

(continued)

DATA	CATEGORY	DESCRIPTION	WEBSITE
National Survey of Substance Abuse Treatment Services	Provider survey	This survey is conducted by the Department of Health and Human Services: Substance Abuse and Mental Health Services Administration and collects information from all facilities in the United States that provide substance abuse treatment services.	https://www.datafiles.samhsa.gov/study-series/national-survey-substance-abuse-treatment-services-n-ssats-nid13519
National Survey on Drug Use and Health	Population survey	This survey is conducted by the Department of Health and Human Services: Substance Abuse and Mental Health Services Administration and collects information on the use of illicit drugs, alcohol, and tobacco and on mental health issues and their effect on the health of civilian, non-institutionalized individuals 12 years and older.	https://www.datafiles.samhsa.gov/study-series/national-survey-drug-use-and-health-nsduh-nid13517
Panel Study of Income Dynamics	Population survey	This panel study, conducted by the University of Michigan: Survey Research Center, is the world's longest running panel study and has over 50 years of data on family economics, demographics, and health.	https://www.icpsr.umich.edu/icpsrweb/DSDR/studies/37142/versions/V1/datadocumentation
Population Assessment of Tobacco and Health	Population survey	This longitudinal study is conducted by the National Institutes of Health: National Institute on Drug Abuse on the use of tobacco and its effect on health of individuals.	https://www.icpsr.umich.edu/icpsrweb/NAHDAP/series/606
Practice Pattern of Young Physicians	Provider survey	This study, conducted by Georgetown University, interviewed physicians about medical practices in which they worked during the past month, the number of hours spent providing patient care, and the number of patients seen in the past week.	https://www.icpsr.umich.edu/icpsrweb/HMCA/studies/02829/version/1/datadocumentation
Robert Wood Johnson Foundation Employer Health Insurance Survey	Population survey	This study, conducted by RAND, collected information from employers and employees about health insurance.	https://www.icpsr.umich.edu/icpsrweb/HMCA/studies/02935/version/2/datadocumentation

(continued)

DATA	CATEGORY	DESCRIPTION	WEBSITE
Study of Women's Health Across the Nation (SWAN)	Population survey	SWAN is a multisite, longitudinal, epidemiologic study designed to examine the health of women during their middle years.	https://www.swanstudy.org/swan-research/data-access
Survey of Income and Program Participants	Population survey	This is a longitudinal survey conducted by the U.S. Bureau of the Census to study income, wealth, and poverty in the United States and its effect on well-being.	https://www.census.gov/programs-surveys/sipp/data/datasets.html
Treatment Episode Dataset: Admissions	Provider survey	This survey is conducted by the Department of Health and Human Services: Substance Abuse and Mental Health Services Administration and collects information on all admissions to substance abuse treatment programs by individuals 12 years and older.	https://www.datafiles.samhsa.gov/study-series/treatment-episode-data-set-admissions-teds-nid13518
Treatment Episode Dataset: Discharges	Provider survey	This survey is conducted by the Department of Health and Human Services: Substance Abuse and Mental Health Services Administration and collects information on discharge of individuals 12 years and older from substance abuse treatment centers.	https://www.datafiles.samhsa.gov/study-series/treatment-episode-data-set-discharges-teds-d-nid13520
Washington Post Nutrition and Health Poll	Population survey	This survey is conducted by the *Washington Post* and asked respondents about their diet and nutrition and their health and well-being, including access to medical services.	https://www.icpsr.umich.edu/icpsrweb/ICPSR/studies/09359/version/1/datadocumentation

13

GLOSSARY

3D maps: 3D maps is a feature in Excel° 2016 and beyond to visualize location data on maps. It is accessed through the "Insert" tab in Excel.

Add-in: Add-in is a feature that needs to be activated in Excel to provide additional functionality in Excel. Some add-ins may need to be downloaded and then activated in Excel.

Alpha value: Alpha value is the probability of failing to accept a null hypothesis when it is true. It is also referred to as the "level of significance" and is usually set at 95%.

American Public Health Association (APHA): The APHA was founded in 1872 to advocate for public health and provide public education to improve community health as well as campaign for health departments at federal, state, and local levels.

Analysis ToolPak: Analysis ToolPak is an add-in that needs to be activated to provide additional functionality for a variety of statistical analysis and functions in Excel.

ANOVA: The analysis of variance (ANOVA) is a statistical test used to determine if there is a statistically significant difference between the means of three or more independent categories.

Array formula: Array formula is a special formula in Excel whose output appears in a range of contiguous cells. After the arguments of the array formula (e.g., frequency) are entered, to get the output to appear in a range of cells, hold down and simultaneously press "CTRL," "Shift," and "Enter" keys.

Area chart: An area chart provides a comparison of how categories have changed over time and includes a proportionality comparison by using the area under the line.

Availability sampling: Availability sampling is a nonprobability sampling approach where elements of the population are included in the sample because of being convenient for research. This approach to sampling is also referred to as "convenience sampling."

Bar chart: Bar charts depict data in horizontal bars and are useful for comparison of how individual categories have changed. These horizontal bars are especially useful when the category names are long.

Bin values: Bin values are the cutoff points for data in Excel that are used for computation of frequencies for a data distribution. The cutoffs provide a range of data values for which the frequencies or counts are computed.

Bubbles: Bubbles in 3D maps in Excel is a method to visualize underlying data through bubbles that are displayed on maps.

Categorization: Categorization in qualitative analysis is the process by which text responses are classified or coded.

Centers for Medicare and Medicaid Services (CMS): The CMS is part of the Department of Health and Human Services and oversees the Medicare and Medicaid programs.

Central tendency: Central tendency measures the midpoint of data and values. Common measures of central tendency are mode, median, and mean.

Claims data: Claims data are data generated for the management of payments for health services provided by healthcare providers and facilities.

Clinical data: Clinical data are data generated by healthcare providers and facilities in the process of delivering patient care.

Cluster sampling: Cluster sampling is an approach to statistically random sampling that is done in stages. For instance, in the first stage a random sample of states is generated and then in the next stage a random sample of hospitals within the state is selected. Cluster sampling is usually used to balance the geographical spread of a sample and still have a random sample.

Columns: Columns in 3D maps in Excel provide a visualization of underlying data using columns that are represented on maps.

Column charts: Column charts represent data on variables and are especially useful to show changes in categories of data over time.

Combo charts: In combo charts, two or more different chart types with different scales are brought together in the same figure.

Commission on Accreditation of Healthcare Management Education (CAHME): Established in 1968, CAHME is an interdisciplinary group of educational, professional, clinical, and other health sector organizations devoted to quality improvement of education for healthcare management and administration professionals. It has established accreditation standards for graduate healthcare management education in the United States and abroad.

Communication domain: Communication domain is a collection of identified competencies that cover application of different aspects of oral and verbal communication.

Competency models: Competency models are a collection of different sets or domains of topical areas that facilitates assessment of application of skills defined for a degree, a function, or a job.

Composite measure: A composite measure is a measure whose value is computed as a combination of values of two or more variables.

Confidence interval: A confidence interval is a range that is computed from sample data such that we have confidence (usually 95%) that the true population value of the data lies in this range.

Convenience sampling: Convenience sampling is a nonprobability sampling approach where elements of the population are included in the sample because of being easily available for research. This approach to sampling is also referred to as "availability sampling."

Correlation: Correlation is a measure of strength of linear relationship between two variables. This strength is measured through correlation coefficient that ranges from +1 to −1 with very strong relationships closer to 1. In this coefficient, the negative sign indicates an inverse relationship between two variables. Note that "correlation" does not mean "causation."

Cost data: Cost data are charges generated by healthcare providers and facilities in the process of delivering patient care.

County Health Rankings: An initiative funded by The Robert Wood Johnson Foundation in partnership with the University of Wisconsin's Population Health Institute, the County Health Rankings provide annually updated data from a variety of sources on socioeconomic, demographic, and health at the county level.

Critical thinking domain: This is the set of competencies that assess application of systematic and rigorous review and analysis processes.

Cross-sectional data: Cross-sectional data are data that are collected only at one point in time from a sample.

Dashboard: A dashboard is a compilation of figures and graphs that provide at-a-glance information on a phenomenon.

Data aggregation: This is a summation or addition of values of a variable.

Data array: A data array is a range of data in a worksheet.

Data elements: Data elements consist of level of measurement, descriptive statistics, and frequency distribution. These data elements guide selection of how the underlying data are best presented through appropriate tables, figures, and graphs.

Descriptive statistics: Descriptive statistics is a range of measures that summarize the values that a variable takes on. These measures typically include central tendency, dispersion, skewness, and kurtosis. Descriptive statistics are also referred to as "summary statistics."

Dispersion: Dispersion measures variability in data. Common measures of variability are range, variance, and standard deviation.

Document grouping: Under document grouping, instead of using the actual words in text responses, the key ideas are used for clustering. Document grouping is an approach to text-clustering analysis in Excel using the MeaningCloud Add-in.

Doughnut chart: In a doughnut chart, data are displayed using doughnuts which are especially useful to show the part to the whole relationship for two or more series of data.

Ecological fallacy: Ecological fallacy occurs if group-level data are used to make inferences about individuals.

Electronic health records (EHR): EHRs are computerized charts on patients that include medical information as well as clinical work flows associated with the patients.

Epi Info™: Epi Info started in 1986 as a desktop operating system (DOS) program and has rapidly evolved into a user-friendly Windows'-based comprehensive suite for quantitative analysis, visualization (including mapping capabilities), and reporting tools in the public domain. This suite is used by public health practitioners, students, and researchers across the world for designing small disease surveillance systems.

Excel: Excel is a spreadsheet program within the Microsoft' Office Suite that is designed to allow users to interact with data for analysis and visualization (charts as well as maps). Using additional features that are activated through add-ins, Excel is useful for qualitative analysis as well.

Factfulness: This is the relaxing habit of carrying opinions that are based on solid facts and reliable data.

Fixed panel: A fixed panel is a form of longitudinal data where data are collected from the same sample at different points in time.

Funnel chart: A funnel chart depicts data from highest to lowest and thus works well with sorted data.

Gapminder: Founded in 2005, Gapminder is an independent Swedish Foundation that serves as a fact tank that produces free teaching resources to make the problems of the world better understood through reliable statistics.

Geographical data: Geographical data are data that have location (GPS coordinates, address, city, county, state, or country) included in the data.

Genomic data: Genomic data cover the basic biology behind the sequencing of DNA, RNA, and epigenetic patterns that help to personalize treatment and medicines for individual patients.

Health Cost Coverage and Access (HCCA) Index: The HCCA Index draws upon related dimensions of access to health professionals and facilities, health insurance coverage, and cost of healthcare to develop an index that is a composite of these dimensions and is scored from 1 to 100 for easy interpretation.

Health systems informatics: Health systems informatics is the bringing together of a transformative bundling that processes data on providers, facilities, and patients.

Heat map: Heat maps in 3D maps in Excel are a visualization of underlying data to show intensity or density using a map.

Hospital Consumer Assessment of Healthcare Providers and Systems (HCAHPS): HCAHPS is a standardized patient satisfaction survey that is required by the Centers for Medicare and Medicaid Services of all hospitals in the United States. This survey contains patient rating of nine topics: communication with doctors, communication with nurses, responsiveness of hospital staff, pain management, communication about medicines, discharge information, cleanliness of the hospital environment, quietness of the hospital environment, and transition of care.

Hypothesis testing: Hypothesis testing is the use of test statistics with a probability distribution to determine which of the two competing alternatives are likely to be true. The failure to reject any competing hypothesis is based on established levels of statistical significance, usually 95%.

Independent observations: Independent observations occur when data are not collected repeatedly from the same sample.

Information management domain: This is the set of competencies that assess application of how data are managed and transformed for specific purposes that aid decision-making.

Institute of Medicine (IOM): The IOM was a division of the National Academies of Science, Engineering, and Medicine, collectively referred to as the National Academies. The National Academies are private, nonprofit institutions that provide independent and objective analysis to inform policy-making on health. On March 15, 2016, IOM was renamed as the Health and Medicine Division.

Interactive Advertising Bureau (IAB): IAB is a classification of terms and words that are used for text analysis in Excel through the MeaningCloud Add-in.

International Press Telecommunications Council (IPTC): IPTC is a classification of terms and words that are used for text analysis in Excel through the MeaningCloud Add-in.

Interval variable: In a variable measured at the interval level, the values of the variable are meaningful in terms of the distance between variables having significance. Thus, a value of 5 as compared to a value of 1 can be stated as being four intervals distant from each other.

Level of measurement: The level of measurement of a variable refers to the scale that is used for measuring the variable. The four scales are: nominal or categorical, ordinal or rank, interval, and ratio.

Line charts: Line charts depict data as lines and are useful for comparing data in different categories over time.

Longitudinal data: Longitudinal data are data that are collected at two or more points in time.

Meaning analysis: Meaning analysis is a component of common approaches to qualitative analysis that focus on understanding what is implied in the responses being analyzed.

MeaningCloud: MeaningCloud is a downloadable add-in that works within Excel to aid qualitative analysis.

Missing values: Missing values occur when one or more records or variables in a dataset do not have a recorded value.

Mixed methods: Mixed methods in research are a hybrid of qualitative and quantitative methods with an intentional focus on one of these methods.

Multiple linear regression: Multiple linear regression is a regression model that uses a straight-line goodness of fit between two or more independent variables and one dependent variable.

Multiple R: The Multiple R is also known as the "correlation coefficient" and is a measure of strength of linear relationship between two variables. This strength is measured through a correlation coefficient that ranges from +1 to −1 with very strong relationships closer to 1. In this coefficient, the negative sign indicates an inverse relationship between two variables. Note that "correlation" does not mean "causation."

National Center for Health Statistics (NCHS): The NCHS is a Center within the Centers for Disease Control and Prevention (CDC). It is charged with coordinating the collection of vital statistics (births, deaths, etc.), provider surveys, as well as registry for diseases such as cancer.

Nominal variable: In a nominal or categorical variable, number values categorize only the variables and no mathematical computation is possible with the values that this variable takes on.

Nonprobability sampling: In nonprobability sampling, the chance or probability of an element from the population being selected is not known in advance of the research.

Normal distribution: In approximately normal distribution, the skewness and kurtosis values are between −2 and +2 and the mean and median are very similar.

One-tailed: A one-tailed test of hypothesis is used to test an alternate hypothesis that is either greater than or less than a certain value.

Ordinal variable: In an ordinal variable, number values are used to rank only the variable values and thus it is possible to assess only those values which are higher or lower than other values of the variable.

Patient-generated data: Patient-generated data are data created or collected from patients, family members, and caregivers related to a medical concern.

Patient preferences: Patient preferences are how patients evaluate different treatments and outcomes and decide which treatment or outcome is in their interest.

Pattern analysis: Pattern analysis is the identification of repetition in a relationship or concept in quantitative or qualitative analysis.

Performance management domain: This is the set of competencies that help to assess application of skills tied to assessing data on progress (or lack thereof) across the input to outcome continuum.

Personalized medicine: Personalized medicine is the customization of medical treatment to the unique characteristics of a patient.

Pharmaceutical data: Pharmaceutical data refer to data on pricing, quantity, dosage, or outcomes related to the use of medicines.

Pie charts: Pie charts display data using pies and are especially useful in showing the relationship of part to whole.

Pivot chart: Pivot charts in Excel are used to visualize summary data from pivot tables to aid analysis of comparisons, patterns, and trends.

Pivot table: Pivot tables in Excel are used on raw data to summarize, analyze, explore, and present summary data in tabular form. Summary data in pivot tables can also be visualized using pivot charts.

Population: In statistics, population refers to the entire or total set of observations or subjects that are being studied.

Population health: Population health is the health-related outcomes that are found in a set of individuals who are defined to be served by a health entity. Population health is not the same as public health.

Population value: Population value uses the entire dataset (not just a sample) of values of a phenomenon for computation.

Power maps: This is a feature in Excel 2013 and earlier to visualize location data on maps. It is accessed through the "Insert" tab in Excel.

Predictions: Predictions are made based on regression (single or multiple) equations by replacing independent variable(s) by specific values of independent variable(s).

Probability distribution: A probability distribution provides the chance of occurrence of a test statistic.

Probability sampling: Under probability sampling, the chance of an element or a member of this population being selected in a sample is known prior to the study and is nonzero.

Problem-solving domain: This is the set of competencies that help to assess the application of skills related to identifying approaches that are used to find solutions to issues that hamper correct application of processes.

Production of tour: In 3D Maps in Excel, once the visualizations using the scenes and tours have been completed, the story or tour is then finalized and produced either as slides (for print) or video (for multimedia).

Purposive sampling: Purposive sampling is an approach to nonprobability sampling where the entire sample is selected based on certain unique characteristics such as insurance status, rural/urban, patients with cancer, and so on.

Python: Python is a high-level general-purpose programming language that has a wide range of applications in statistics and web development.

Quality improvement (QI): QI is the systematic and continuous application of processes designed to make measurable progress or betterment on an identified problem or issue.

Qualitative analysis: Qualitative analysis is the range of approaches to analysis of nonquantitative or textual data from interviews, observations, open-ended responses, reports, and the like to identify patterns, relationships, and meaning.

Qualitative methods: Qualitative methods in research are used when specific events and actions are thought to result in particular outcomes.

Quantitative analysis: Quantitative analysis is the range of approaches to analysis of numeric data using mathematics and statistics to compute estimates, test hypotheses, and undertake comparisons.

Quantitative methods: Quantitative methods in research are methods used when variations in independent variables are followed by variations in dependent variables, holding everything else constant.

Quota sampling: Quota sampling is an approach to nonprobability sampling where the sample selected takes cognizance of special characteristics (rural/urban, race, gender, etc.) of subsets of the population and ensures that these are represented in appropriate numbers in the sample.

R: R is an open-source programming language for statistics and visualization.

R^2: R^2 is a measure of the goodness-of-fit of a regression model and is interpreted as the percent of variation in a dependent variable explained by the regression model.

Radar: A radar is like a spider web and shows how three to seven categories of data are represented in the total.

Rapid cycle research (RCR): RCR is the process of identifying and framing problems and step-wise application of analytical methods that are appropriate to the identified problems.

Ratio variable: In a variable measured at the ratio level, the ratio of the numbers is meaningful. Thus, the values of 4 and 1 for a ratio variable denote that the ratio between the two values is 4:1.

Reductionist fallacy: Reductionist or individual fallacy occurs if data collected at the individual level are analyzed to make inferences about a higher level such as family or group.

Regression: Regression is a statistical approach to analysis of the relationship between two or more variables that helps to explain the amount of variance in a dependent variable explained by the independent variable(s). The relationship between variables can be linear or nonlinear.

Repeated cross-sectional data: Repeated cross-sectional data are a form of longitudinal data that are collected from different samples at two or more points in time.

Research design: Research design includes the methods (qualitative/quantitative/mixed), data (longitudinal or cross-sectional), and unit of analysis for a study or research.

Research question: Research question is the statement of a problem in a way that is amenable to research and analysis.

Sample: In statistics, sample is a subset of the entire or total set of observations or subjects that are being studied.

Sample estimate: A sample estimate uses a subset of data on a phenomenon to compute a statistic.

Sampling: Sampling is the process of identifying a subset of a population for purposes of research. Two broad approaches to sampling are probability and nonprobability sampling.

Scatterplot: A scatterplot uses dots to visualize the relationship between two sets of data.

Scene: Scene in 3D Maps in Excel provides a single visualization of a table with location variable and another variable of interest.

Sentiment analysis: Sentiment analysis categorizes text data as positive, negative, or neutral as well as whether they convey agreement or disagreement. In Excel, sentiment analysis is used within the MeaningCloud Add-in.

Simple random sampling: Sample selection under simple random sampling is statistically random, not haphazard. Random number generator, a formula in Excel, can be used for simple random sampling from a list.

Snowball sampling: Snowball sampling is an approach to nonprobability sampling where the sample is built up based on recommendations from initial respondents who identify other respondents for inclusion in the study.

Social determinants of health: Social determinants of health are all factors in a person's living, learning, working, and aging environment as well as healthcare options and governmental policies.

Social media model: Social media model for text classification is available in Excel through the MeaningCloud Add-in. This uses common social media nomenclature for classifying text from social media.

Single linear regression: This is a regression model that uses a straight-line goodness-of-fit for the relationship between one independent and one dependent variable.

Spatial analysis: Spatial analysis is the analysis of data that includes a location (address, city, county, state, or country) variable. In Excel, spatial analysis is undertaken using Power Maps.

SPSS: SPSS initially was branded as Statistical Program for the Social Sciences and is now developed as a statistical software for business and research problems.

Standard deviation: Standard deviation is a measure of dispersion and shows how spread out the data are.

Standard error of the mean: The standard error of the mean is the standard deviation of a sample divided by its sample size.

Stata: Started in 1985, Stata is a statistical software for data science.

Statistic: A statistic is any computation that is based on a subset of data on a phenomenon.

Statistical Analysis System (SAS): Founded in 1966, SAS developed as a statistical software before branching into business analytics and services together with its core statistical software capabilities.

Stratified random sampling: Under stratified random sampling, sampling is statistically random and uses different strata such as rural/urban, insured/uninsured, and so on to create bands within which statistically random sampling would be applied.

Student t-test: The Student's t-test assesses the significance of the difference in average or mean value of data for two groups of small samples. This test is also referred to as "the t-test."

Summary statistics: Summary statistics is a range of measures that summarize the values that a variable takes on. These measures typically include central tendency, dispersion, skewness, and kurtosis. Summary statistics is also known as "descriptive statistics."

Systematic random sampling: Under systematic random sampling, the first sample is selected using a statistically random process such as a random number and the subsequent elements of the sample are selected using a preset interval such as every 10th, 20th, ith member.

t-Test paired two-sample mean: This t-test is done when we are interested in the results of a pre- and posttest that is undertaken with the same sample.

t-Test two-sample mean assuming equal variance: This t-test assesses the significance of the difference in average or mean value of data for two groups of small samples under the assumption that the population underlying these two categories has equal variance for the variable that is being tested.

t-Test two-sample mean assuming unequal variance: This t-test assesses the significance of the difference in average or mean value of data for two groups of small samples under the assumption that the population underlying these two categories have unequal variance for the variable that is being tested. Variance of the two categories is considered unequal if the standard deviation of the two categories differs by a factor of 2.

Tableau: Tableau is a visual analytic software that helps people see and understand data.

Text classification: Text classification is the process of categorizing or coding text responses. In Excel, text classification is undertaken through the MeaningCloud Add-in.

Text clustering: Text clustering is used to analyze text responses to identify words or categories around which the text responses center. In Excel, text clustering is used within the MeaningCloud Add-in.

Topic modeling: Under topic modeling, words within the text responses are used for analyzing clustering of responses. Topic modeling is an approach to text clustering used within the MeaningCloud Add-in in Excel.

Topic extraction: Topic extraction is used to analyze text responses to identify underlying themes and ideas. In Excel, topic extraction is used within the MeaningCloud Add-in.

Tour: Tour in 3D Maps in Excel brings together visualizations (or scenes) of a location variable with another variable of interest around a common theme or story that relates to the purpose behind the visualization using 3D Maps.

Tree map: A tree map depicts data to provide a comparison of each category to total.

Trendline: A trendline in a scatterplot is a line of best fit for the data. This line of best fit can be linear or nonlinear in order to be the line of best fit for the underlying relationships.

Triple Aim: The Triple Aim is a framework developed by the Institute for Healthcare Improvements that uses population health, patient experience, and per capita cost of care to optimize health system performance.

Two-tailed: A two-tailed test of hypothesis is used to test an alternate hypothesis that is equal to a certain value.

Unit of analysis: The unit of analysis is the primary level at which analysis of data is planned based on the research question. This may be at the individual, family, group, city, state, or country level. The unit of analysis may or may not coincide with the unit of data collection.

Unit of data collection: The unit of data collection is the primary point at which collection of data for a research occurs. The unit of data collection could be an individual, family, group, city, state, or country. The unit of data collection may or may not coincide with the unit of analysis.

Variable: A variable takes on different values and is not constant.

Visualize: Visualize is the process of picturing data through a graph or figure that helps to answer the question posed.

Vital statistics: Vital statistics are data on life events such as births, deaths, marriage, and divorce.

Years of potential life lost (YPLL): YPLL is a measure of untimely mortality and provides an estimate of the average number of years persons would otherwise have lived if they had not died.

Z-Score: A Z-score is the number of standard deviations that a data point is from the mean.

Z-Test: A Z-test is a statistic used to test if there is difference in two means from large sample sizes.

INDEX

Note: Page numbers followed by *f* and *t* indicate material in figures and tables, respectively.

CPSIA information can be obtained
at www.ICGtesting.com
Printed in the USA
BVHW012332260922
648019BV00009B/74

9 780826 150271